We're Pregnant!

How to Receive
God's Cure
for Infertility

Dianne Leman

We're Pregnant! How to Receive God's Cure for Infertility

Published by: fox and hare publications

ISBN 978-1518642890

Scriptures taken from:

The Message. Copyright © by Eugene H. Peterson 1993, 1994, 1995, 1996, 2000, 2001, 2002. Used by permission of NavPress Publishing Group.

NASB — NEW AMERICAN STANDARD BIBLE®, Copyright© 1960,1962,1963,1968,1971,1 972,1973,1975,1977,1995 by The Lockman Foundation. Used by permission.

NLT — Holy Bible, New Living Translation, copyright 1996, 2004. Used by permission of Tyndale House Publishers, Wheaton, Illinois 60189. All rights reserved.

ESV — English Standard Version copyright 2001 by Crossway, a publishing ministry of Good News publishers. Used by permission. All rights reserved.

Cover Design: Katie Goulet
Interior Design: Jody Boles

http://www.dianneleman.com/

fox and hare publications

Dedication

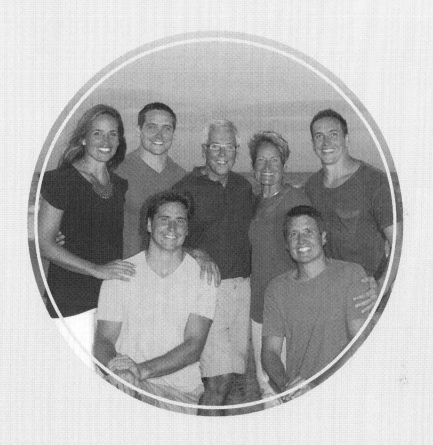

To my five "impossible" children:

Julie, Cory, J.D., J. and A.J.

Thank you for making me
the joyful mother of children

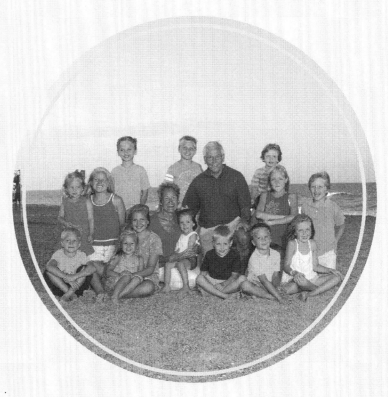

Dianne and Happy Leman with their grandchildren, 2016

Table of Contents

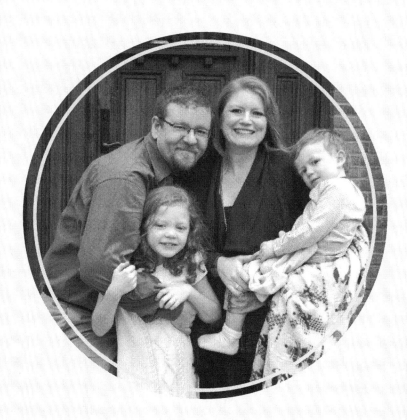

Beau, Heather, Stella and Samuel Crandall

Preface

God has many more babies to be born, and yours is one of them. Now, that is a bold statement. How can I say that? After almost 40 years of interacting with and praying for couples who longed for a baby but were unable to conceive, I am more convinced than ever that this is true. God does have many more babies to be born and if you are reading this, I truly believe that one of those babies is yours. God is the Ultimate Father, and babies are His absolute delight. He desires to bring many more beautiful human beings into the world and He chooses to use us, His very own image bearers here on earth.

Life, human life, is so very precious. And, human life is far more valuable, far more enriching, than all the fame, fortune, and fun the world has to offer. Family is God's incredible gift to us. That is why your heart aches if you are struggling with infertility. That is why your body cries to be cured and to carry a child. God is the Giver of Life and He actually trusts us to love, care, and nurture that life. Many of you have sought cure after cure for your infertility, only to be disappointed once again. If this all sounds a bit crazy to you, that's okay. I know this promise and proclamation are outlandish, but I do believe this is true. No matter where you are on your spiritual journey, or even if you are not on a spiritual journey of any kind, I invite you to read and to consider this as truth: God has many more babies to be born, and yours is one of them.

Even though I do not know you or know your own personal pain and heart-ache, I do know God wants to fill your home with lots of laughter and lots of laundry. He wants to delight you with sloppy kisses and sloppy kitchens. He longs to help you love unconditionally and learn unashamedly that in His eyes, you are the perfect parent for your child. He is a Father. He designed family. This is what He does best and He chooses to do it through us, His beloved sons and daughters here on earth.

God created human beings; He created them godlike, reflecting God's nature. He created them male and female. God blessed them: "Prosper! Reproduce! Fill Earth! Take charge!" (Genesis 1:26-27 MSG)

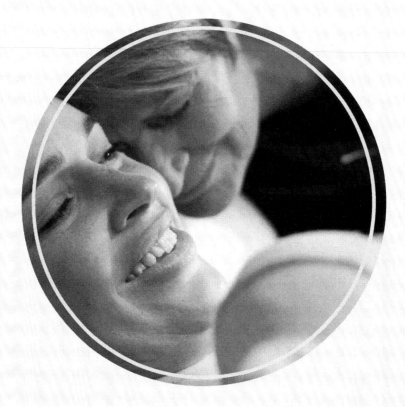

Dianne, rejoicing with daughter Julie and newborn Magdalena Marie

I do not know your specific heartache, but I do know that I long to weep with you through your journey of infertility. My desire is that my experience will spark hope in your hearts and one day, we will rejoice together. Thank you for being courageous!

Introduction

Yes, There is Hope!

"We're pregnant!"

"We're pregnant!" These were the words I longed to shout with joy at my husband. I imagined the jubilant scene over and over in my mind. We would laugh, cry, and hug one another with delirious delight. I rehearsed our impending celebration dinner at Papa Del's, our one-of-a-kind local restaurant, where I would reach for another piece of the deep-dish pizza and giggle about "eating for two." Together we would devise the cleverest way to tell our eager parents that finally, a grandchild was on the way. And, of course, I would pull out the list of beloved boy and girl names I had labored over and we would narrow it down to the top four. Ecstasy would abound! Our dream had at last come true. After three long years of frustrating infertility, we would relish this celebration because: "We're pregnant!"

Bad News Again

But, at 4:37 p.m. on this cool autumn day in October 1976, that dream turned into a nightmare once again. I had just heard the nurse at our local hospital say over the phone, "I am sorry, Mrs. Leman. Your pregnancy test came back negative." Choking back hot tears, I sank onto the sofa, overwhelmed with sorrow, confusion, anger, and despair. "Why?" I screamed. "Why can't I get pregnant? Unmarried fifteen-year-olds don't seem to struggle. What have I done wrong? I try to live a good life. Why isn't my body responding? We have done everything the doctors told us to do."

My husband and I had both been so sure that this month I was finally pregnant. I had a strange aversion to coffee. I had been extra tired. Our mid-cycle timing had been perfect. That morning I had eagerly dropped off my first morning urine to be tested at the lab. All day it was hard to concentrate on teaching my first grade students as I waited to race home at four o'clock and listen for the call. Now, we faced another month of tedious "trying." I was suffocated with hopelessness.

The Shame and Hopelessness of Infertility

"Why, God? Why can't I have a baby? Why is this happening to us? What do we need to do?" Like a helpless rag doll, I surrendered again to the sobs that consumed my entire being. This was such a feared, yet familiar, darkness. The pain of infertility was brutal and all-consuming to my soul. The shame of infertility stole every ounce of my self worth. Was there any hope that I would ever conceive a child?

You Are Not Alone

Because you are reading this book, I assume you can identify with some of my experience. The pain and hopelessness of infertility is quite universal. More than any other time in documented history, women and men are battling infertility. While both men and women can have a fertility problem, current statistics (Centers for Disease Control and Prevention, 2015) show there are about 6.7 million women in the US and over 70 million worldwide who struggle with infertility. You are not alone in your pain or your mercurial hope.

I Want to Give You Hope

But I want to do more than comfort you with the patronizing sentiment of "I know how you feel." I actually do not know how each of you feels deep down in your aching heart. But I do know I want to give you hope. Fresh hope. I want to say to you, "Yes, there is hope." And, I want to share with you our story of how we were filled with hope, cured of infertility, and now enjoy a vibrant, albeit chaotic, family tribe of 28 and counting. This is our story, but it can be your story, too.

How do I know? I have learned many valuable lessons over the years that have convinced me how much God loves each person, including *you*. You may be a person who does not know God or maybe you do not even know He exists. Maybe you are of another faith or maybe you are an atheist. You may be a committed disciple of Jesus or a lukewarm Christian. No matter where you may be on your personal spiritual journey, I am confident of God's love for you. This is a bold statement and it is okay if it seems untrue to you. It took me time to grasp this life-changing truth. I desire to impart God's love to you in a way you can experience for yourselves. The same God who loves me, loves you.

God's Desire

I am also confident that it is God's deep and even passionate desire to give you children. Again, this is a truth I had to learn. I had many mixed-up beliefs about God, His character, and His will. Now, I believe God is eager to bless every couple with children. This may sound audacious or presumptuous to you.

It certainly did to us at one time. You may be asking, as we did, "If God is so eager to give us a child, why can't we get pregnant?" My husband Happy and I were told there was a slim to no chance of our ever conceiving our own child. We both had serious medical issues. We had exhausted the available treatment options. Our cries to God went unanswered. We certainly had no idea God wanted to do miracles for us or anyone else.

Then, all of that changed. Not only did we receive God's cure and healing from infertility for ourselves, but we also went on to share with over five hundred couples who, like us, received God's cure and the blessing of children. Many of these couples likewise shared with other infertile couples and rejoiced as they, too, were cured and had children.

God Does Not Play Favorites

Contrary to popular belief, God wants to bless every couple and He does not play favorites. He is truly a loving Father, and He designed the human race to enjoy family life. Again, this may be foreign to your beliefs, as it was at one time to ours. That's okay! I will share with you the many important lessons we learned on how to receive God's cure for infertility and His gift of children.

No matter the severity or impossibility of your current diagnosis, I encourage you to read this book. I am aware of the courage that may take. I am well aware of how dangerous hope can be. I often wanted to protect my heart from even daring to hope again when we were in the throes of treatment and trying. I invite you to open your hurting heart just a bit. I take this very seriously. I know how fragile I was when we struggled month after desperate month. It was often excruciating to lay down my armor of self-protection, crack open my heart, and hope again. I do not want to give you false hope. I do not want to add more disappointment to your shattered emotions. *I want to give you fresh hope.*

I have found that God's love is a love that never fails, even in the darkest times. This was a startling, life-changing discovery for me.

God's Love Does Not Fail

So, I come gently, yet confidently, to you. I speak to you now as a mother, a grandmother, a pastor, and most of all, as one who knows the love of God. I have found that God's love is a love that never fails, even in the darkest times. This was a startling, life-changing discovery for me. It may be impossible or difficult for you to comprehend this in your current situation. Again, that's okay. He loves you now, even if you do not know it or feel it or find it hard to believe. I want to help you receive the baby I believe God has for you. I want to help you hope again. One of my greatest joys is hearing the news: "We're pregnant!"

Lessons Learned

For over 35 years I have witnessed God's amazing cure for infertility and His blessing couples with the children they had lost hope of ever having. While there are no magic formulas or "get pregnant quick" tricks, there are many solid, true, and practical lessons God has taught others and me through the years that will help you receive the cure and the children you so desperately want. Whether you learn and apply these lessons alone or join with others, I believe you will receive the help you need. Many of the lessons I have learned have come from joining with others.

Journeying Together

We like to gather a small group of us to meet with a struggling couple. We spend about an hour sharing and then praying with them for God's miracle. Even though I am a pastor, it is not necessary to be in any kind of formal ministry to apply the lessons I share. Most of the people in our groups are ordinary men and women who love to help others and have often been helped themselves. When we pray for couples, we trust Jesus with them and for them.

Every Couple is Unique

Right now, we are praying for 15 couples who are waiting to experience the miracle of pregnancy. Each situation is different. Each couple is unique. Yet, their pain is similar. Some of these couples have tried for many years to get pregnant, while others have only been trying for a year. Some are young and healthy, while others have the difficulty of being over 40 years of age. A number have the heartbreak of multiple miscarriages or serious medical conditions. Some simply have what the medical profession calls "undiagnosed infertility." Many wrestle with jealousy, anger, and despair.

Many couples have tried countless remedies and complex procedures. The possibilities offered today—like potent fertility drugs or intrauterine insemination (IUI)—are only a click away, and the desire for a baby has often driven couples to try it all. Quite a few couples have exhausted their insurance, their savings, and their medical options. They are often at the end of their rope because they know studies show only 50 percent of infertile couples actually have a child, either on their own or with medical intervention. They sometimes come to us with caution, skepticism, and even the cynicism that infertility can so subtly breed.

Sharing Pain, Sharing Prayer

As a prayer team, we share in the pain of each infertile couple. Our hearts are stirred with compassion as we hear their stories, and we weep together. Many have endured multiple rounds of IVF (In Vitro Fertilization), surgery, or other procedures. We assure them we are grateful to medical science for all the advances in treating infertility, and we are not opposed to such.

However, we also are bold to share that we believe in the power of prayer and the goodness of our God. We relate our conviction that it is God's will to bless them with children. We encourage them that while God can and does use medical intervention, He also can and often does perform unexplainable miracles. Often it is a combination of medical help and miracles from God that result in a healthy pregnancy.

Over the two years of writing this book, we have rejoiced with 19 couples who conceived and gave birth in response to prayer. Again, some of them had medical intervention, while others did not. All received prayer. These couples join the hundreds of others who, over the past 35 years, have received children after we prayed for them.

Others' Stories Encourage Us

Because I want to encourage you, I share many of their stories in this book. Sometimes the details in a couple's story are very private, so I have chosen to change their names, except for my own daughter, Julie, and her husband, Mike. The Appendix stories, written by the couples themselves, reveal all the actual identities, unless otherwise noted. I want these stories to bring you hope. I am confident there will be many more expectant couples as a result of this book.

More Than Coping

Much of what has been written about infertility from an emotional or a spiritual perspective gives couples tools to cope with the pain and devastation of infertility. I am grateful for that comfort and consolation. However, my emphasis will be how to *hope*, not cope. Coping can help, but it does not heal. I want to give you fresh hope. At the same time, I want to be sensitive to the fact that hope can be hard and scary. I want to specifically highlight the hope God brings to couples who have experienced the sickness of heart that the deferred hope of pregnancy brings.

Promises in God's Word

The Bible, which I believe to be God's Word, has a verse written by King Solomon thousands of years ago. These words capture what so many of us have endured:

> *Hope deferred makes the heart sick, but a dream fulfilled is a tree of life (Proverbs 13:12).*

Month after month of deferred hope of ever having a child, truly makes a heart sick. Every negative pregnancy test wounds an already damaged heart. Hope that doesn't deliver what it promised can destroy. But I believe God wants to fulfill your dream of having a child. I believe He longs to bless you with new life. I believe He wants to heal your heart and body. Time and again I have seen God do what He promises in the Book of Psalms.

> *He [God] gives the barren [infertile] woman a home, making her the joyous mother of children. Praise the LORD! (Psalm 113:9).*

God makes the infertile woman "the joyous mother of children." Yes, and there is so much joy!

A Joyous Journey

But usually the joy is not without some tears. Pregnancy often does not happen instantaneously. There is an uncharted journey ahead for you, a journey filled with a few challenges, some sorrow, and abundant joy. There are also very clear truths for you to consider and to embrace. There are lessons for you to learn and practical steps you can take. Ultimately, this journey leads to joyous victory for you. This is a victory made extra sweet by the triumphant defeat of the seeming impossible. When you endure the tension and trauma of a tough contest, your joy overflows all the more. I believe you can be the joyous mother of children. I believe your joy can, and will, overflow.

Celebrating Together

As I write, it is summer—my favorite time of year. I am in a three-story vacation home overlooking the vast Atlantic Ocean on the Outer Banks of North Carolina. This early in the morning all is quiet except for the sound of gentle waves lapping against the shore. However, as the sun rises, the stillness will be punctuated with joyful noises of children's laughter, newborns' hungry cries, and playful banter among adults and children alike. With our five children, our five wonderful in-laws, and a houseful of rambunctious grandchildren, there is never a dull moment during this special one-week vacation to the Eastern shore. Sunny summer days are filled with building sand castles, surfing on boogie boards, capturing crazy crabs, and endless swimming in the ocean and pool alike. Papa Hap (aka Grandpa) has already left to make the daily run to Duck's Donuts, where he will purchase three dozen of the most delicious, decadent donuts for the entire crew.

Energized with gratefulness, I head to the still quiet kitchen to pour my first cup of steaming French roast coffee. My heart bursts with joy and singing. I am reminded again of the words spoken by the prophet Isaiah:

> *Sing, barren woman, who has never had a baby. Fill the air with song, you who've never experienced childbirth! You're ending up with far more children than all those childbearing women (Isaiah 54:1-2).*

"Sing barren woman, who has never had a baby?" At one time that seemed like a cruel admonition to me. "You're ending up with far more children than all those childbearing women." That sounded impossible and maybe even a bit insane. But I discovered it was true. We ended up with far more children than we ever dreamed of.

We are so thankful for our family. But, more important for you to know, we ended up with hundreds (probably thousands as we lost count!) of children whose births were somehow tied into our story.

Our Story Can Be Your Story

We are so thankful for our family. But, more important for you to know, we ended up with hundreds (probably thousands as we lost count!) of children whose births were somehow tied into our story. This is a dream designed by God, and I believe this book will enlarge it even more. I do not believe it is by accident that this book is in your hands. As you read these chapters, I invite you to prepare your heart to fill with fresh hope.

What's Ahead

There are nine chapters, divided into three parts: Our Story, Your Struggles, and Receiving God's Gift of Fertility. Each chapter concludes with Important Truths for Your Journey and Suggested Action Steps. In addition, there are four Appendices with stories and resources to encourage you on your journey. With love and tenderness, I share our story, the lessons we have learned, others' stories, and actions you can take—all to give you hope. Yes, I believe there is hope for you. I believe our story can be yours, too.

With Affection and Hope,

Dianne Leman
(or "Manna Di"—the name bestowed by our oldest grandchild, Lily Anne Leman)

> *I pray that God, the source of hope, will fill you completely with joy and peace because you trust in him. Then you will overflow with confident hope through the power of the Holy Spirit (Romans 15:13).*

PART I

Our Story

Our story is filled with lots of plans (gone awry!), pains, and promises. Then there were the many surprises (which were often not understood initially!) and the many solutions to our problems that had not even been on our radar. And while every story is different, I believe there are a few similarities in our story that will bring you hope.

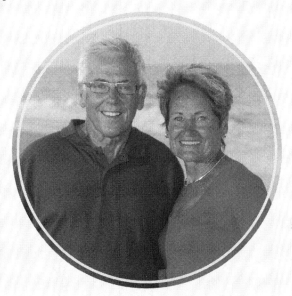

Dianne and Happy Leman, 2016

You are a human being, made in the image of God, and you have much worth and value. God the Father loves you deeply and has an amazing destiny for you, which I believe, includes a family. It's okay if these ideas are unfamiliar to you and maybe even difficult to believe. God does not play favorites, and He is eager to fill your life with good things. I desire for these chapters to encourage you that God is writing a good story in your life. I believe the next leg of your journey can be an exciting adventure of faith (risky to be sure!), hope (which takes fresh courage), and joy!

Plans, Pains, and Promises

"My life plan was disrupted."

I came to the University of Illinois in 1969, eager to experience the freedom and excitement of college life. I was raised in a loving Christian home, but was not at all interested in pursuing God. Classes, new friends, parties, a Greek sorority, and late-night escapades soon filled my days. Before I knew it, I fell in love with a handsome senior, Happy Leman. Like me, he had abandoned all interest in God, church, and religious life of any kind. Together we planned our future, where he would make a million dollars before he turned 30, I would fulfill my dream of a doctorate in education, and one day we would have a home full of children, laughter, and love.

Getting Married, Meeting Jesus

Happy and I married on a hot, summer day in August 1971. Although a Christian pastor performed our marriage ceremony, we had no intention of ever embracing the Christian faith. We actually pledged to one another that we would never become Christians. That fall, we began our new life on the campus, crazy in love, drenched with happiness, and content without God.

Well, one month into our blissful marriage, I met Jesus. I was reading a historical fiction novel where one of the characters had a relationship with Jesus that was intimate, real, and inviting. Before I realized what was happening to me, I began to weep and say, "I want to know *that* Jesus." I had known religion. I had known church. I thought I knew God. Hadn't Happy and I agreed we wanted no part of Him? What was happening to me? I was a university student who was not given to emotional outbursts about God. But, here I was, encountering a God who had much better plans for my life than I had ever dreamed up. I was experiencing the love of a God I had never really known. And the name of this God was Jesus.

Of course, I had to tell Happy what had happened to me, sitting on that green sofa reading a random book at 405 N. Mathews Street in our honeymoon home on a warm September afternoon. While initially surprised and somewhat dismayed, Happy soon had his own encounter with Jesus. Together we joined a local church and experienced a fresh hunger and desire to know God more.

Time for a Baby

Life was good as Happy launched a successful financial planning career and I began teaching special education students in the public school while working on my graduate degree. Happy was on his way to making that first million, we bought our first home, and it wasn't long before we decided it was time to start a family. I had several issues with my cycle through the years, but being on the Pill had wiped those out. I no longer had irregular cycles or heavy bleeding or strange and painful cramping. We were confident we would conceive as soon as I stopped taking the Pill. We started making plans for the year ahead.

However, month after month, I was not pregnant. My periods did not really resume, so it was very confusing every 30 days or so. I always thought I was pregnant, would take my early-morning urine in to be tested at the local clinic (way before home tests!), and wait for the call from the nurse to give me the results. As the months dragged on with no sign of pregnancy, my hope waned. No periods. No pregnancy. No hope. I was filled with mounting despair.

Did God care about our struggle and mounting hopelessness? During these first three years of our infertility struggle, I did not really know the answer to that.

Trying and Trouble

After a full year of trying, I made an appointment with my doctor. He listened to our experience, did a few tests, and prescribed drugs to start my cycle. We started to faithfully chart my temperature, but there was never any sign of ovulation. We took fertility drugs but again, no sign of ovulation or menstruation. Year Two passed with more tests, more drugs, more remedies, and more discouragement. The doctor was running out of options and we were running out of money.

When will we be able to join the growing group of happy pregnant couples who surround us at work and church? I wondered. When will we be the ones shouting, "We're pregnant!"? I was losing all hope.

Did God care about our struggle and mounting hopelessness? During these first three years of our infertility struggle, I did not really know the answer to that.

Confusion About God's Plan

I was confused about God's plan for my life. Was I destined to only enjoy my students and not have children of my own? I loved my job as a special education teacher in the public schools. My days were filled with the wonder of watching five-year-olds read a word for the first time and seeing their absolute delight. My room was a beautiful mess of spilled paint, cookie crumbs, and smelly gerbil cages. We laughed. We cried. We were captivated by the joy of learning. But my heart yearned for my own child to hold, to teach, to love. Was this just my selfish desire or did God want this too for me?

What is your will for our lives, God? What do you want for us? Is your plan for me to be a second mother to these children and not have any children of our own? If so, please tell me and I will stop hoping. But I never heard God speak.

Other people told me to be content with being a teacher. They said God wanted this for me. Teaching was a worthy calling in life. I had the chance to impact many children. My head spun with confusion about God's plan for me. Meanwhile, my desire to bear a child only grew stronger and more overwhelming. My physical condition grew more frustrating and hopeless. I needed a miracle.

Bad News

After multiple rounds of drugs to start my nonexistent menstrual period and other drugs to release healthy eggs, I had neither sign of a period nor any indication of ovulation, let alone ovulation of viable eggs. The next step in our treatment for infertility was a laparoscopy. In gynecology, doctors use diagnostic laparoscopy to inspect the outside of the uterus, ovaries, and fallopian tubes in diagnosing female infertility. Usually they make one incision near the navel and a second near the pubic hairline. I was put under anesthesia and received an incision near my navel. My doctor then had visual access to my reproductive organs to determine how best to proceed in helping us conceive.

The results of the laparoscopy were not encouraging. They discovered I was missing one fallopian tube and one ovary. In addition, my uterus was infantile and nonfunctioning. No wonder I had no menstrual periods. I did have one healthy fallopian tube and ovary, but the ovary was not releasing eggs. My treatment options were very limited. We had already tried fertility drugs to prompt the ovary into action, and they had not worked. I was filled with despair once again.

Questions

Questions flooded my weary brain. What did we need to do to have a baby? Why was this happening to me? I was a disciple of Jesus and tried hard to live a good life. Had I committed some terrible sin? Was God angry with me? Did He or did He not have power to help me? Why couldn't I know what He wanted? He seemed a million miles away and totally silent. Where could I get answers to these haunting questions?

Frustrated and bewildered, I decided to now search the Bible in hopes of finding some answers to my questions on the printed page. After all, our medical options were evaporating. Our money could not buy us what we so desperately wanted.

Fresh Insights

Since I had been a disciple of Jesus for several years, I was accustomed to reading my Bible on a daily basis. Frustrated and bewildered, I decided to now search the Bible in hopes of finding some answers to my questions on the printed page. After all, our medical options were evaporating. Our money could not buy us what we so desperately wanted.

Interestingly, although I had been raised in a Christian home and had always read the Bible stories about Jesus, I was amazed at what I discovered in my fresh search. I discovered that God not only cares about the sick, but God also *cures* the sick. The Bible is filled with many accounts of Jesus curing sickness and physical ailments. Why, everywhere Jesus went, He healed people. So much of Jesus's ministry was focused on healing all kinds of people from all kinds of sicknesses and diseases.

Story after story recorded in the Gospels of Matthew, Mark, Luke, and John tell of Jesus having great compassion on the sick and miraculously healing them. I even discovered that He cured a woman who had bleeding (menstrual) problems. Mark, a disciple of Jesus, tells this story:

> *A woman in the crowd had suffered for twelve years with constant bleeding. She had suffered a great deal from many doctors, and over the years she had spent everything she had to pay them, but she had gotten no better. In fact, she had gotten worse. She had heard about Jesus, so she came up behind him through the crowd and touched his robe. For she thought to herself, "If I can just touch his robe, I will be healed." Immediately the bleeding stopped, and she could feel in her body that she had been healed of her terrible condition. Jesus realized at once that healing power had gone out from him, so he turned around in the crowd and asked, "Who touched my robe?" His disciples said to him, "Look at this crowd pressing around you. How can you ask, 'Who touched me?'" But he kept on looking around to see who had done it. Then the frightened woman, trembling at the realization of what had happened to her, came and fell to her knees in front of him and told him what she had done. And he said to her, "Daughter, your faith has made you well. Go in peace. Your suffering is over" (Mark 5:25-34).*

This so encouraged me. This woman had a serious condition in her reproductive system of constant bleeding for 12 long years. She had spent all her money on doctors and had actually gotten worse. I identified with her. I sensed her physical and emotional pain. I admired her courage for seeking out Jesus in a male-dominated culture that forbade women from traveling alone. I loved how Jesus honored her and made her well. I wondered how she had such powerful faith.

Could I Be Cured?

I trembled with excitement at the thought that such a thing could happen to me, too. Somehow I knew if Jesus were here right now, He would cure me. I imagined touching His robe and being cured, just like the woman in this story. Of course, I knew that Jesus was not here on earth now like in the story, but I had a strange sense that He wanted me to be cured of my infertility. I couldn't wait to ask my pastor about Jesus and healing. Although my church never talked about physical healing, I thought perhaps this was just an oversight. I made an appointment to meet with my pastor and share my excitement and my questions. Did I dare hope that Jesus had a miracle for me?

No Miracles Today

My newfound hope quickly turned to familiar despair when my pastor firmly but gently informed me that Jesus was no longer doing miracles today. Such things were only done when Jesus was alive on earth, he said. *But,* I silently cried, *there are still so many who need miracles, including me.* Such healings had "passed away," he told me with dogmatic authority. He spoke as one who knew his Bible and who knew Jesus far better than I did. Miracles had just vanished? Why? Why did Jesus stop doing miracles? It seemed so unfair.

Searching the Bible

In spite of my disappointment, I continued my search in the Bible. I really found a friend in King David, writer of many of the Psalms. I loved how he poured out his heart to God. When I stumbled on Psalm 37 I was greatly encouraged:

> *Delight yourself in the Lord; and he will give you the desires of your heart (Psalm 37:4).*

Yes! God actually wanted to give me the desires of my heart. My greatest desire was for a child. Now, if I could only figure out how to delight myself in the Lord. Then, as the Scripture said, God would grant me my desire.

Bursting with eager excitement, I shared my newfound revelation with my husband, Happy. We were on this journey together, but because I was the one most emotionally connected to the problem, I was more intent on finding a solution. He listened with patience and a slight look of pity. "Di, I don't want to dampen your enthusiasm, but that passage is in the Old Testament. That no longer applies to us today. That promise is not for us."

My face fell. My shoulders sagged. Suddenly, my Bible was not only confusing, but also seemed totally irrelevant for today. If Jesus no longer did miracles and if the prayers of the Old Testament were invalid in the 21st century, what part of the Bible could I believe? What part was for today and for me?

More Confusion and Anger

How would I ever know God's will? He seemed so very far away. I was more confused than ever. Maybe life was just a matter of "que sera, sera": *what will be, will be.* Maybe I was destined to be a special education teacher for the rest of my life. And, maybe "my children" would be those in my classroom. As much as I loved teaching and loved my students, I was so saddened by this fate. I wanted to bear my own child. I wanted my belly to swell with the life of another human being. *Oh God,* I pleaded. *What is Your will for me? What is Your plan for my life?*

I knew as a "good Christian girl" that was the proper question. Yet I battled anger towards God. Didn't He care at all about what I wanted? He seemed so unjust, so unloving, and so unkind. A slight hardness crept over my wounded heart. I could do this without God. God's silence and my encounters with the naysayers dampened my initial excitement that maybe, just maybe, Jesus still cured people today as He did in Bible days. Now my heart turned to maybe, just maybe, there was a brilliant doctor somewhere who had a medical miracle for us.

Seeking a Medical Miracle

This was 1977 and, unlike today, I could not just Google for more information on fertility treatments. After doing some time-consuming research, I finally located and called an infertility specialist, Dr. M., at Northwestern Hospital, near Chicago. In 1977, infertility doctors and treatment options were limited. My husband and I felt quite lucky to have secured an appointment with Dr. M., and we were prepared to pay the substantial costs. It would be worth it, right? We informed our local doctor that we were pursuing other opinions, and confidently left his office, ignoring the doubtful look of empathy in his eyes.

We arrived at the prestigious hospital after a harried three-hour drive into the city. We were filled with fresh anticipation and headed right to the obstetrics department. We bounded into Dr. M.'s wood-paneled office for our initial consultation. His walls were plastered with happy photos of smiling babies. I surmised each infant was the result of his expertise in treating infertility. I already imagined our baby's picture joining his collage. Meanwhile, I felt the familiar, albeit nervous, trust in this expert's ability to solve our infertility problem rise in my heart. I felt hope awakening once again. I allowed myself to think that soon, yes very soon, I would be pregnant.

Dr. M. checked our records and then proceeded to perform a variety of tests on me. Although my husband had been diagnosed with a lower sperm count, his condition was not addressed at this time, since I had the more serious issues. We were both satisfied with the efficiency and expertise of the entire staff. We loved the positive attitude and confidence exuded by all.

Several hours later, we were on our way home, where we would wait for a call to alert us to return for our test results. The nurse cautioned that it could take several weeks. That seemed like an eternity to me. But I knew anything was worth a wait if it resulted in a baby. What I did not know was what would ensue as we waited for Dr. M.'s report. Unlike the past, this turn would send us on a whole new journey.

"Did You Know God is Still Doing Miracles?"

During that next week, my husband was working in his downtown office when a casual friend stopped by. While Steve (not his real name) worked in the same building, he and Hap were only slightly acquainted. Hence, his bold question was quite surprising.

"Did you know that God is still doing miracles?" he asked.

Startled, my husband warily replied, "No, but actually, we need one. Tell me more." Hap did not believe in miracles, or at least that was what both of us had been taught. But Steve was a smart guy who, like us, had graduated from the University of Illinois. He was not at all a religious fanatic. Yet, Steve believed God still did miracles? He had Hap's attention.

Steve explained that he was just an ordinary Christian whose life had been impacted by this new discovery that God did miracles. Then he invited Hap to attend a meeting in a few weeks where a speaker would teach on miracles and pray for people to be cured. This was all very unusual and intriguing at the same time. Why was Hap given an invitation to a miracle meeting from a man he barely knew at the exact time we desperately needed our own miracle? More bewildering was how did Hap find himself, a logical man with an MBA, actually interested in this invitation to a miracle meeting? And all this occurred in the fourth floor office of a downtown financial planning business in the middle of an ordinary March day. What was going on?

Skeptical, But Intrigued

When Hap told me about this conversation, I was somewhat skeptical but intrigued. Wasn't this what I had hoped was true when I read the Bible and asked my pastor about Jesus curing people? But my pastor said God did not do miracles anymore. I thought I had settled this. We were going to get our miracle from Dr. M. Or were we?

I agreed we would mark our calendars to go. What harm could it do to attend a miracle meeting? We might suffer the playful derision of our friends who, like us, did not believe in such things. But, that was not enough to keep us from going. My head and heart argued a bit, but I somehow knew I needed to go to this meeting. After all, I, more than anyone else, knew I needed a miracle.

Meanwhile, we had our upcoming appointment with Dr. M. Maybe we would discover that I did not need a miracle from God. Maybe Dr. M could work his medical magic on my messed-up body.

"You Will Get Bad News. Don't Worry."

Right before we were to leave for Northwestern, Hap returned from a business trip with an unusual announcement. "While I was driving home today," he said, "I heard God speak to me."

"What?"

I was incredulous. Neither of us believed that God still spoke in that way. We knew we had the Bible and that was the way God communicated with people now. We did not believe a person could actually hear the voice of God. Of course, we were having a hard time hearing Him there, since so much of the Bible seemed irrelevant to us. I did not know what parts applied now or were no longer relevant. I had to admit that although I had a Master's degree in Education from the University of Illinois, the Bible was more confusing to me than ever. This was especially true in the past few months as I made a more earnest attempt to understand it. Oh, sure. I could do a Bible study with the best of them. And I had notebooks to prove it. However, when it came to actually knowing the will of God and hearing Him through His written Word, I was really struggling.

> He went on to explain that this was not an audible voice of God but was instead a very strong thought in his mind that he knew was not his own thought but was God speaking. Well, that was interesting.

"So what exactly did God say to you?" I asked, full of doubt.

"God told me we are going to get very bad news in Chicago this week," he said, "but we are not to worry. Everything is going be all right."

He went on to explain that this was not an audible voice of God but was instead a very strong thought in his mind that he knew was not his own thought but was God speaking. Well, that was interesting. I wasn't at all convinced that this was God speaking. It seemed too nebulous and subjective to me. However, I figured we would soon discover if the first half of this message from God were true. Our appointment with Dr. M was just a few days away.

"You Will Most Likely Never Conceive Your Own Child"

After making the distant trek to Northwestern Memorial Hospital, we rode the elevator to the upper floor. We waited what seemed like an eternity before the nurse called our name. Since this would be a report of test results and not the usual doctor visit, we were ushered into Dr. M.'s personal office and not into an examining room. After exchanging cordial hellos, we sat down, eager to hear his findings.

"Well, Mr. and Mrs. Leman," he began slowly, "it looks like you are good candidates for adoption. There is a 90-plus-percent chance that you will never conceive your own child. As a matter of fact, our test findings align with your previous results. In addition, we have detected a rather large growth in the uterine area—about the size of an orange—and we are recommending surgery for this. There is a good chance we would do a complete hysterectomy when we open you up. We would need your permission to go ahead and do that while you are under anesthesia."

What could be worse news than that? This was absolutely horrible, horrible news. No chance of conceiving our own child? Adoption, as wonderful as that is, our only choice? Possible hysterectomy? This was a death sentence to our dream of bearing our own child. But, strangely, for the first time in the three long years of hearing one bad report after another and of responding with gut-wrenching weeping, I did not feel devastated. I did not cry. Instead, I calmly replied, "Thank you very much, Dr. M. We will talk this over and get back to you."

But, something inside me knew we would never be back to this place. We had indeed received the bad news that God had told Hap we would hear. So, the first part of God's message had been true. Did that mean the second half—that we were not to worry, all would be okay—was also true? Had God really spoken to us, personally? Was God assuring us that He heard our cries for a child? Was this what it felt like when God communicated to me—a fresh sense of peace that He really did have our backs? Hope began to bubble within me.

Daring to Hope Again

Did I dare let hope rise in my heart again? That was dangerous. I wanted to guard my heart. Keep hope at bay. Protect my fragile emotions. But a tiny flame of hope had already begun to burn within. In just a matter of days, that tiny flame would burst into a veritable fire. We were about to meet the God who still does miracles. We were about to experience the Fire Himself, God's Holy Spirit.

Important Truths for Your Journey

* God seeks us, even when we are not one bit interested in Him.
* God loves us and has amazing plans and promises for us.
* Often, our pains open us to God and His solutions.
* God may send people across your path who can radically change your life.

Suggested Action Steps

* Reflect on your life and look for where God may have been seeking you.
* Open your heart to embrace unfamiliar concepts, such as miracles.
* Begin to listen for "nudges" or strong impressions that may be God speaking to you, and act on what you hear.

Surprises and Solutions

"I like control. No surprises, please."

It was a warm spring day in May 1977, and our Midwest world was bursting with new life, chirping birds, and fresh, vibrant colors all around. We were alive with cautious excitement and slight apprehension as we drove the two hours to Indianapolis, both wondering what lay ahead. We were on our way to the meeting to hear about this God who does miracles. Would we come home with our own miracle and new life? Would our struggle with infertility finally be over? My heart said *yes* but my head shouted *no way*.

Different Music

The huge convention center was packed with thousands of people. The atmosphere was festive, expectant, and friendly. Gingerly we made our way through the crowd and found two open seats just as the music began. Immediately, we were assaulted with the realization that this was no ordinary church music, although it was a religious gathering. We were immersed in what appeared to be a rock concert, not a church service. There were no hymnbooks, no organ or piano, and no hymns. Instead, on a large stage was a full band—complete with drums, guitars, keyboard, saxophone, and a multitude of singers. All around us, people sang, raised their hands, shouted, and even jumped up and down. This was considerably different from our non-instrumental worship service at the church we attended. It really was quite surprising to two conservative churchgoers! While we were a bit overwhelmed and somewhat uncomfortable, we could not deny the unmistakable joy gushing forth from thousands of participants.

Strange but Interesting Message

While this was all new and awkward to us, nothing could dampen our interest in the slated speaker. We were eager to hear him share about this miracle-working God. After 45 minutes of group singing, the speaker finally came to the stage and began teaching. However, instead of teaching on healing or miracles, he taught from the Bible about the Person of the Holy Spirit. It was all very interesting, but quite strange to us. We knew little about the Holy Spirit, although we had been Christians for five years and active in our church and reasonable students of the Bible. We knew some Christian leaders warned people to beware of excessive emphasis on the Holy Spirit. As the speaker continued to talk enthusiastically about the Holy Spirit, we shifted in our seats and nervously thumbed through our Bibles.

Our discomfort intensified as the speaker encouraged people to "get baptized in the Holy Spirit" just like the early Christians. What if this was not really a biblically correct idea? What if we were on the verge of serious deception? At this point, we weren't sure why we had made this trip, but decided we would discuss what we had heard and consider our response.

Next Steps

As we drove the two hours home, we agreed we were both pretty disappointed that we did not learn about the God who does miracles. After all, wasn't that why we went? And, we did not even receive prayer from the speaker or anyone else to cure our infertility. Maybe, we thought, this was all a mistake.

Nevertheless, the more we talked, the more we realized we did want to consider the Holy Spirit and possibly "be baptized in Him." Really, what did we have to lose? We were at the end of our rope and both felt an inner tug to risk. We were not clear what it all meant or how to go about it, and we were both nervous to "speak in tongues," as the speaker said the Bible showed sometimes happens when one is baptized in the Holy Spirit.

I knew that I wanted to keep this nice, neat, and under our control. I did not want to do anything fanatical or crazy. We were both smart, college-educated professionals who lived a normal, quiet Christian life. All we wanted was to receive a cure for our infertility and finally start our happy family. I did not realize at the time that God wanted so much more for me, for us. He wanted to enlarge our view of Him and to increase our experience of His love and power. He wanted to introduce Himself to us as the God who still does miracles. He wanted us to be baptized in the Holy Spirit.

There, in the quiet of a moonlit May night, I knelt down and simply asked Jesus to baptize me in the Holy Spirit. In spite of my carefully made plans, I did this without having everything figured out.

Surprised by the Spirit

We were both somewhat scared, but we were also filled with an inner calm as we arrived home late that night. We planned to do a Bible study and discuss with others what we had heard. We knew a good night's sleep would help us think more clearly. However, despite being dead tired and emotionally drained, I couldn't sleep. My mind was filled with thoughts of all the speaker had said about the Holy Spirit. I felt a strong urge to get out of bed and head to the downstairs office to think and pray. This was not something I had ever done before, but right after midnight, I stole out of bed while my husband was asleep.

There, in the quiet of a moonlit May night, I knelt down and simply asked Jesus to baptize me in the Holy Spirit. Despite my carefully made plans, I did this without having everything figured out. I had not begun any Bible study to ascertain the truth of this experience. I only knew I wanted to know God more. I knew I desperately wanted and needed a miracle from Him. I also knew I must relinquish my control to His love and trust Him for things I did not understand. I had no sooner asked Jesus to baptize me in the Holy Spirit, when I sensed a bubbling sensation in my stomach and chest and I began to speak in a language I did not know. Surprise! All of this happened in just a few short moments and then I got up, went back to bed, and fell asleep.

(See Appendix C for instructions on praying to be baptized [filled] in the Holy Spirit and an explanation of the gift of tongues.)

Surprised by the Bible

When I arose the next morning after being baptized in the Spirit, I picked up my Bible to read a few chapters as I had done almost every day for the past five years. I was not prepared for what happened next. It was as though scales had completely dropped off my eyes. I could now read the Bible with understanding. Before, I had had so much confusion. I had not known which parts of the Bible still applied to me today. I was confused about Jesus and His miracles; I thought those no longer occurred. Now I knew that Jesus was indeed still doing miracles. My first revelation happened as I was reading that morning in the Book of Hebrews:

> *Jesus Christ is the same yesterday, today, and forever (Hebrews 13:8).*

The words jumped off the page. My heart raced. My mind reeled. I exclaimed, "So Jesus *is* the same today. He *is* still doing miracles. I can ask Him to cure us and give us a baby right now." It all made so much sense and seemed so real. This Holy Spirit was opening my eyes and my heart to truths about Jesus! I devoured the Gospel of Mark and discovered what a compassionate, powerful miracle worker Jesus was. I knew then and there He would cure me of my infertility. But I had no idea how it would take place.

Fresh Confidence in God

Of course, I quickly shared with Hap about my midnight encounter with the Holy Spirit, and he was eager to pursue his own experience. Several days later, he too received a baptism in the Holy Spirit, and we opened our Bibles to discover more surprises about the God who does miracles. We were truly on this journey together, partners in our marriage and in our desire for a family. While we certainly did not have everything figured out, we had a fresh confidence that God did have the solution to our problem, that He had a cure for our infertility. With the baptism of the Holy Spirit, the Word of God had come alive to us. Our minds were beginning to comprehend what we previously had struggled to understand. We were delighted and surprised over and over again to discover new things about God.

Through our Bible study, we discovered that God is 100 percent good and that He really loves all people. We saw that God is eager to cure all physical problems, including infertility, that He wants families to have children, and He is ready to give us all this just by asking Him. (In the appendices I note numerous Scripture passages and books that are relevant to this discussion.)

These were surprising—no, shocking—truths to us. At times, we felt silly, even stupid, for believing them. We struggled with why we were not cured if God was so good, so powerful, and so willing to give children. However, since we had no other solution, we chose to believe that God was ready to give us a child. We decided we would ask Him to cure us and bless us with a baby.

Almost eleven months after specifically praying for healing and for our baby, I still had no signs of being cured or of pregnancy. I daily battled doubt, but I asked God to help my unbelief and show us how to keep trusting Him.

So Much More to Learn

The date was June 1977. Of course, I thought we would be pregnant within a week. That did not happen. Almost eleven months after specifically praying for healing and for our baby, I still had no signs of being cured or of pregnancy. I daily battled doubt, but I asked God to help my unbelief and show us how to keep trusting Him.

God had so much to teach us. We had asked for our healing and for a child to be conceived. God wanted us to believe He heard us and loved us, and that we had received our healthy conception, although we could not see this. We knew so little about trusting God. We were quite used to logic, reason, figuring things out, and being in control. This trusting God was a whole new experience for these two college-educated know-it-alls. We learned many valuable lessons about trust during this time. But, in the process, my patience wore thin; my hope diminished to almost nothing. It was difficult every day to choose to trust a God I could not see with my own eyes and to believe He had answered our prayer.

Adoption Choice

Then, on April 21, 1978, my husband and I received a call from the local adoption agency that jolted our world. The agency director told us that we would most likely be receiving a newborn in several months. Earlier in our quest for a child, we had completed all the paperwork, home inspection, and paid the initial fees required of those wishing to adopt. We had both long forgotten this after we learned of God's will to cure us and bless us with our own child. The waiting list for adopting newborns was quite lengthy, and it often took years before one's name moved up the list. Ours was now on top. We were being offered the chance to become parents in just a few months.

My heart pounded. Was this God's answer to our prayers? We both knew God has a huge heart for adoption. He loves the orphan. He calls us His adopted children. We had witnessed what a blessing adoption was in other families.

As I asked God about this, knowing we had to give a prompt response to the agency, I heard God say, "Why are you considering adopting this baby?"

That surprised me. However, I quickly responded, "God, I know You are for adoption." He replied, "Yes, that is true. But, I asked you, why are you adopting this child?"

Of course, we cannot hide the truth from our all-knowing God. Why was I even considering this option? I pondered this question. Then, it rose up in my heart and I haltingly responded, "Because . . . I guess . . . I really do not think You are going to come through with our own pregnancy."

I was somewhat shocked that came out the way it did. But I know it was the truth. Left to myself, I probably would have said something like "I think You are giving us a blessing" or "I want to be open to Your ways" or something other than an outright indictment of God's character! Instead I said, "I don't think You are coming through."

That is like saying, "I do not think You are faithful, God. I do not think You keep Your promises, God. I doubt You, God." Yikes! Our doubt was exposed.

I knew what we had to do. My husband was in total agreement. We wrote a letter to the adoption agency explaining that we would soon be having a baby. We asked them to please remove our name from their list of couples wanting to adopt a newborn infant. We then placed the letter in the mail on April 22, 1978. We had acknowledged our doubt to God. We asked him to fill our hearts again with faith in Him.

Fresh Faith in Our Hearts

That is exactly what He did for me: a renewed gift of faith entered my heart that day—faith from God that allowed me to just rest and trust Him. We had heard God. We had obeyed His gentle voice. He truly loved us and was for us. He was teaching us how to walk with Him, how to trust Him completely. Although there were no immediate changes in my physical condition, I had recommitted to trust. Was this easy? No. A thousand times, no! But I knew He was my source of faith and strength.

Three months later, I sweltered in the blazing July sun and battled an ongoing uneasiness. It felt as if something was a bit off in my body. Did I dare return to the doctor after 15 months of no medical attention? Would he chide me for my stupidity in trusting a miracle-working God? I had boldly announced I would not come back until I had my miracle. Now I regretted such brashness. I decided to make an appointment with another obstetrician to avoid any confrontation.

After listening to a description of my concerns, this new obstetrician did an initial exam. "Well, I think you may be premenopausal. I'll do a few other tests to see what's going on." I knew I shouldn't have come! Was I just a fool? While I withered inside, he did a few more pokes and prods. Suddenly he left the examining room without saying a word and he had a bewildered look on his face.

When he returned, he carried a strange-looking instrument and placed it on my belly. "Do you hear that?" he calmly asked. A gentle thump-ity, thump, thump-ity thump sounded in my ears. "Someone is living in you," he quietly announced.

Surprise! Someone is Living in You

When he returned, he carried a strange-looking instrument and placed it on my belly. "Do you hear that?" he calmly asked. A gentle thump-ity, thump, thump-ity thump sounded in my ears. "Someone is living in you," he quietly announced. What? My mind raced out of control. Someone is living in me? That gentle sound was the heartbeat of a baby? Joyous surprise!

Not caring that I was wearing a skimpy hospital gown in a sterile office with a doctor I did not know, I jumped off the table and shouted, "Praise the Lord! Thank you, Jesus!" He smiled a professional smile and said I was already about three months pregnant. He went next door to grab my actual doctor, who hugged me and said, "This is truly a miracle from God."

We can't know for sure, but I am almost positive that the day we told the adoption agency we would not need their baby, April 22, 1978, was the night we conceived our first son. Of course, we did not know I was pregnant until July, three months later. My body was not menstruating at all. I was being extremely cautious about any bodily pregnancy clues. Now it was confirmed that God had cured me and a baby was on the way. That evening, Happy and I danced and shouted, "We're pregnant!" Then we headed off to Papa Del's Pizza to celebrate God's surprising, miraculous solution.

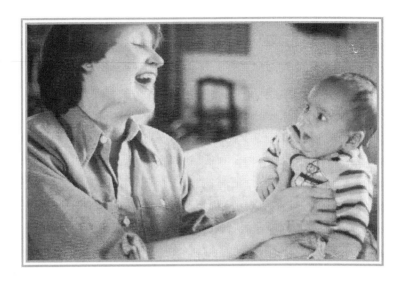

Surprise Son, Surprise Ministry

For the next six months, I made sure I ingested nutritious meals and panted my way through thousands of kegel exercises. Most of all, every day I thanked God for this amazing gift of a miracle baby. Jonathan David Leman made his grand appearance on a cold, snowy January 26, 1979, after just six hours of natural labor.

Jonathan's birth thrust us into a new way of life in more ways than one. Only nine months after his birth, I discovered I was pregnant with our second son, Andrew. This convinced us I was indeed healed through and through. No more growths. No more malfunctions with my menstrual cycle. My body was healed and whole. And within ten years, we had two more sons and one daughter, all conceived naturally and with ease. Our hearts overflowed with thanksgiving.

We eventually left our careers to enter the ministry as we watched God do miracle after miracle and people were eager to know and experience more. One of the greatest surprises was God's plan for us to pass on His cure for infertility and watch Him bless hundreds of families with children.

We believe you are one of those families. We are aware some of you are struggling to hold on to any hope at all. Please continue reading. Part II will address some of the struggles you may be facing right now. Then, Part III will provide you a way forward giving you help on how to receive God's cure for your infertility. There are also a variety of helpful resources in the appendices. All of this is so you, too, can shout, "We're pregnant!" and we will celebrate with you. God's surprising solution is for you, too.

Important Truths for Your Journey

- God loves to surprise us with new and sometimes strange new experiences and truths.
- God is still doing miracles today.
- God may unexpectedly bring people into your lives that speak important truths.

Suggested Action Steps

- Consider learning more about the Holy Spirit; Read a recommended book or pray to be baptized in the Spirit (see Appendices C and D).
- Investigate what the Bible has to say about miracles; Read the Gospel of Mark.

PART II

Your Struggles

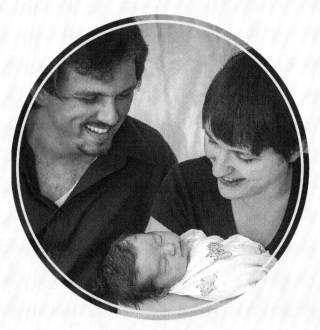

Tim and Sarah Schiro
Baby Margaret joined brother Isaiah

Every couple has unique struggles, and each is marked by very real pain. This can be actual physical pain or deep emotional, spiritual, or relational pain. These chapters explore three painful dilemmas: "I don't know if I even believe in God"; "It is impossible for us to get pregnant"; and "There is nothing medically wrong, but we just can't conceive." In addition to lessons I have learned, actual couples share their stories here and in Appendix B to help you navigate your pain and receive new hope.

Chapter 3

God Believes in You

"I don't know if I even believe in God."

He shifted his weight and tugged at his shirt with awkward nervousness as he waited for me to exit the church sanctuary. Despite obvious anxiety, his face reflected the humility I have come to admire among the many Chinese people who live in our diverse university community. "May I speak with you for a moment, Mrs. Leman?" he asked in broken but understandable English. I could tell this took courage. After all, he was a young foreign man speaking to an older American woman in a language he did not know well, in an unfamiliar setting. I smiled warmly to relieve the tension and replied, "Of course."

En-Chen introduced himself and his wife, Cheng, and shyly explained that he and Cheng were unable to have a child. They had been married seven years, endured the grief of two miscarriages, and had sought much medical intervention with no cure. He was distraught and discouraged. His wife was desperate. He so wanted her to be happy. He did not know what else to do. "I really do not know if there is a God," he stammered with embarrassment. "And if there is a God," he continued, "I certainly do not know if I believe in Him." Because they had been raised in a country that for many years had forbidden belief, it was understandable that neither of them knew much about God. He went on to say that his wife had recently expressed some faith and had been invited to the church service by an American friend. Someone had told them that we prayed to God for people to be cured of infertility.

"Can you help us?" he whispered. "Would you possibly be willing to pray to God for us to have a child?" He lowered his eyes to avoid my gaze as he shared such an intimate request. My heart filled with compassion for this precious Chinese man. I knew how much God loved him and his wife, even if they did not know Him. I knew how much God believed in them, even if they did not believe in Him. I knew God was very eager to help them, cure them, and fill their empty arms with a child. I assured him a small team of people and I would gladly meet with them for an hour to hear their story and ask God to cure them and give them a child. Thankfulness and relief flooded his face; joy burst from my heart. This was another opportunity to give away what God has given to me—a strong faith in His desire to cure infertility and to give a struggling couple fresh hope— even if they did not know or believe in this miracle-working, all-loving God.

> *Despite what you may have been taught, believed, or experienced, God is real. God is very good, and most important of all, God loves you. He created you. He wants to have a relationship with you. He wants to give good things to you, including a child.*

God is Good and He Loves You

Despite what you may have been taught, believed, or experienced, God is real. God is very good, and most important of all, God loves you. He created you. He wants to have a relationship with you. He wants to give good things to you, including a child. God believes in you even if you do not believe in Him or have no desire to know Him. Yes, God loves you, believes in you, and is delighted to cure you of infertility. But I know how difficult this can be to believe.

We live in a time when many in America and around the world no longer believe in God. We have made many advances in science and technology that have replaced the need and desire to believe in an unseen God. Faith and reason can at times appear to be polar opposites and incompatible. Belief in God seems both unreasonable and unnecessary. God does not seem very real or very nice. Even many who once believed in God have now abandoned that belief.

Misconceptions About God

Others hold on to faith in God, but have confusing beliefs about His character and will. There are so many misconceptions about God that have been perpetrated by wrong teaching, media, and even our own experiences. It is not uncommon to blame God for the bad things in our lives. Even the Bible can give one the idea that God is angry or that God does not really love people. These misconceptions can easily lead people to think God is not for them or is punishing them. These misconceptions can result in a rejection of God or a crisis of faith.

While I always had a basic belief in God, I had no use for Him and thought He was generally distant and usually upset with me. Then I met Jesus. I did not fully realize that Jesus is God, but I have since learned this powerful truth. Getting to know Jesus cleared up much of my confusion about God. I discovered that Jesus is so loving, so full of compassion, and so willing to heal, no matter what disease or condition. I discovered how much Jesus believes in each and every person, no matter who you are, where you have come from, what you have done. Jesus loves you.

Satan is Our Enemy

I also learned that there is another powerful being in the universe—a real enemy named Satan—who hates every one of us and is determined to bring despair and destruction into our lives. For the first five years of my Christian life, I did not know there was a supernatural realm. I did not know angels and demons really existed. I had often thought only the uneducated believed in these and I was so much smarter to not believe in such things.

How wrong I was! I did not know that we have a real enemy named Satan. Oh, I had heard of the devil. However, I did not know he was responsible for sickness and affliction. I was unaware that he is a deceiver, an accuser, and an outright liar. I did not know he wanted to mess up my ideas about the love of God and the power of God and God's desire to give us children.

But God's Word is clear. Satan is the father of lies. Once, Jesus was in a dialogue with some religious men who were opposing Him. He said:

You are of your father the devil, and your will is to do your father's desires. He was a murderer from the beginning, and does not stand in the truth, because there is no truth in him. When he lies, he speaks out of his own character, for he is a liar and the father of lies (John 8:44).

Satan is a liar and the father of lies. Satan and his lies are at the root of many struggles with infertility. This was startling news to me. As I have shared, I was confused about God's role in my life. Did God cause my infertility? That is what Satan told me, sometimes through other people. Did he want me to remain childless for some sovereign reason I did not know? Yes, Satan convinced me that was my lot in life. Was God really a good God? Satan made sure I questioned God's goodness and love for me.

God is Very Good

But ... Jesus showed me so clearly that God is good. Very good. Satan is bad. Very bad. God is indeed large and in charge and the ultimate ruler over all. Yet, there is another player on the field. Even though I was a follower of Jesus and in the church for five years, I was unaware of Satan and his destructive activity. I thought if anything happened to me, it was God's will—good and bad. After all, wasn't God all-powerful? Didn't He control everything? Wasn't He executing a plan for my life? I was just watching it unfold and accepting "what will be, will be." Only after I was filled with the Holy Spirit did I see Satan for who he really is—the liar, thief, destroyer, and perpetuator of infertility.

God Gives Good Gifts

I also saw clearly that God is good—all the time—and the giver of good gifts, including children. Jesus's disciple, John, recorded this comparison spoken by Jesus:

> *The thief (Satan) comes only to steal and kill and destroy. I (Jesus) came that they may have life and have it abundantly (John 10:10).*

Satan is a destructive thief. Jesus wants us to have an abundant life. Jesus believes in me. Jesus believes in you. Jesus came so we could have a life overflowing with His love and gifts, including the gift of children. I had been ignorant of these wonderful truths. I had also been ignorant of the reality of Satan's destructive work in the world. Now I saw clearly the goodness of Jesus and His power over Satan.

When Jesus ministered on earth, everywhere He went He announced that the Kingdom of God had come. He healed all the sick. He demonstrated over and over that the rule of God, the Kingdom, had usurped the rule of Satan. One of the most prevalent and powerful ways Jesus showed that God is the King was by healing the sick and freeing the demonized:

Jesus traveled throughout the region of Galilee, teaching in the synagogues and announcing the Good News about the Kingdom. And he healed every kind of disease and illness. News about him spread as far as Syria, and people soon began bringing to him all who were sick. And whatever their sickness or disease, or if they were demon possessed or epileptic or paralyzed— he healed them all (Matthew 4:23-24).

Jesus healed them all. And He is still doing the same for us.

Jesus's death on the cross, His powerful, victorious resurrection, and His ascension to heaven all assure us that He has ultimate authority in heaven and on earth. This is very important. Everyone and everything must bow to the Name of Jesus. Everything—including infertility.

Jesus Has Authority Over All Satan's Work

Jesus's death on the cross, His powerful, victorious resurrection, and His ascension to heaven all assure us that He has ultimate authority in heaven and on earth. This is very important. Everyone and everything must bow to the Name of Jesus. Everything—including infertility. Infertility is not just a physical and emotional issue with a natural solution ("Take this drug, have this procedure, just relax, have more sex, etc."). There are important spiritual elements that also affect it. Every case of infertility is different, but each struggle often includes a variety of factors, including emotional, physical, and spiritual.

Satan is the Author of Sickness

Satan is the author of sin, sickness, and pain. Satan afflicts people with demons. These are real. These are not figments of the imagination or some silly superstition that only primitive people believe. On the contrary, these are part of a real, supernatural realm that many "intelligent" people do not acknowledge. That was certainly how I thought at one time. When you cannot see something, it is easy to believe it doesn't exist. Because this activity of Satan can affect us in physical ways that are familiar, such as endometriosis or PCOS or blocked tubes, we can think it is just a medical or physical issue. Of course, I do not think that all infertility is a result of demons. That is not what I am saying. But, the supernatural realm is real and right here, and some infertility is directly related to evil influences.

Jesus Defeated Satan

The good news is Jesus has power and authority over all evil and can bring healing where people have been damaged by evil sources. It is important to know God paid a big price to destroy Satan's works, which includes some causes of infertility. Jesus came specifically to demolish the works of Satan. One of the most debilitating works of Satan is infertility, because it stops the reproduction of new life through women. Satan specifically hates women. Jesus came in love to set us free. Jesus defeated Satan through His death on the cross and His indisputable resurrection. The prophet Isaiah tells of Jesus' experience on the cross:

> *Surely our sicknesses he (Jesus) hath borne, and our pains——he hath carried them . . . And by his bruise there is healing to us (Isaiah 53:4-5, Young's Literal Translation).*

Jesus took our sickness, pain, and sin on the cross. When He rose from the dead, He demonstrated that he had won a complete victory over the rule of Satan. The Kingdom of God has come. Eternal life is available. Healing is available. Freedom is available. Fertility is available. Faith in God is real.

Jesus Wants All to Be Cured

Jesus, filled with the Holy Spirit, went about healing the sick and showing us that this is God the Father's will. Our Father, like a good father, does not want any of His children to suffer sickness. He made a way for us to live in health and enjoy an abundant life. He definitely uses medical advances to heal and help and He sometimes needs to address other elements that we may be unaware of. These elements can be hindrances to healing; Chapter Five addresses these in depth.

But It Can Be Confusing

However, it can be confusing when you learn Jesus heals and yet you are not cured. It can be frustrating to see the promises of God and not experience them for yourself. It is perplexing that things are not more automatic. It is easy to blame yourself or wonder if somehow you are not included in God's blessings. Why, God? If You are so good and Jesus dealt with evil, why am I still struggling?

Be Assured

Be assured, God wants to show you how to receive His cure and His blessing. Meanwhile, it is so good to know you can stop blaming God for the hurt, pain, and hopelessness in your lives. You now know Satan is the enemy. You also know God is not cursing you. God is not causing infertility. God is the Healer and the Giver of Life. God loves you and is for you. He wants to bless you with a child. He wants you to know the joy of motherhood.

God believes in you, even if you are still not sure if you believe in Him. He is very aware that some of you are even struggling right now as you read this, because your heart is breaking.

God believes in you, even if you are still not sure if you believe in Him. He is very aware that some of you are even struggling right now as you read this, because your heart is breaking. You got your period again. There is no sign of being cured. If this is God's desire, why isn't it happening? It is okay to ask God your questions and to pour out your heart to Him. He will answer you.

Ask God to Reveal Himself to You

You can ask God to reveal Himself and His love to you. This may come in a dream or from reading the Bible or from reading this book or some surprising way. You will begin to know the truth and this will empower you to start truly trusting Him as the loving Father He is. Jesus especially wants to pour the love of the Father into your heart by His Spirit. This strengthens hope and fights off the shame and fear so prevalent in infertile couples. This is powerful hope from God Himself:

> *Hope does not put us to shame, because God's love has been poured into our hearts through the Holy Spirit who has been given to us (Romans 5:5).*

The Holy Spirit wants you to know and experience the Father's love. Many have had earthly fathers who were less than perfect, sometimes even abusive or absent. This can damage your view of the heavenly Father. This can destroy your faith in God. However, you do not need a perfect earthly father to reveal to you the Father above.

Jesus Himself showed us the Father, and Jesus alone is the Way to the Father:

> *Jesus said to him, "I am the way, and the truth, and the life. No one comes to the Father except through me" (John 14:6).*

This is such Good News! It is very liberating to know my broken, dysfunctional family on earth cannot stop me from being fully loved and accepted by my Father in heaven. Jesus made it possible for me to become a fully righteous, much loved daughter of the Father:

> *But to all who did receive him (Jesus), who believed in his name, he gave the right to become children of God, who were born, not of blood nor of the will of the flesh nor of the will of man, but of God (John 1:12-13).*

When we receive Jesus, we become a brand new person, born from God, His very own child. If you are not yet a child of God and you want to be, you can stop right now and turn to Appendix C and pray the simple prayer of receiving Jesus and all He has done for you.

It's OK to Doubt

Others of you are still uncertain about a relationship with God, and that is absolutely fine. Take your time. This is a very important decision and not one to make in haste. You are on a journey, and even if you are not sure about God, you can know that God believes in you. Some of you are still unsure about the reality of Satan, and about the truth of God's love for you and His desire to cure you of your infertility. Again, that is okay. Please keep reading. Express your doubts. Read some of these passages in the Bible. Open your heart and mind. Your unbelief or skepticism is welcome. This book is for you, too. I believe God has some amazing surprises even for those who are unsure about Him or who do not believe in Him at all. God may surprise you like He surprised En-Chen and Cheng!

"We're Pregnant!"

It was a great day of rejoicing when En-Chen and Cheng ran up to me at church and told me they were pregnant. Music to my ears! We immediately prayed for a full-term, healthy pregnancy, because she had suffered two miscarriages and had much fear about losing this baby. Although there was some sign of physical distress a few weeks later, we prayed and God brought assurance to her heart that all was well. They asked if I would give their daughter her American name. (Chinese couples give their babies Chinese names but may also have an American name.) Months later, I was delighted to welcome and hold their healthy, miracle baby, Piper Elyse. Through this experience, both En-Chen and Cheng came to truly believe in the God who believed in them, even when they were not sure.

Your struggle with uncertainty, skepticism, and unbelief does not stop God's rich love for you. You are made in His image, and He longs for you to reproduce that image and to experience for yourself the joy of children. Keep learning. Take time to think deeply about these things. Examine your unbelief. Be open to the truth that God believes in you. God loves you.

Important Truths for Your Journey

- God is good!
- Satan is a real being and is real bad.
- Jesus has dealt with Satan and brings us freedom and healing.
- God believes in and loves you as one made in His image.

Suggested Actions Steps

- Ask God your questions and listen for thoughts that pop in your head.
- Ask God to reveal Himself to you. Note your dreams or resources that come your way.
- Read the Gospel of John.
- Consider praying to receive Jesus if you have not done so already.

Chapter 4

God Has a Baby for You

"It is impossible for us to get pregnant."

"It is impossible for us to get pregnant," sobbed Maeve. "We just suffered another failed IVF. After my ectopic pregnancy, we thought IVF was our miracle. But now, due to some serious complications, the doctor's prognosis is pretty grim. My husband and I are exhausted with grief. Our anger is at a real tipping point. There doesn't seem to be much medical hope at all. It looks impossible for us to ever have our own child." I put my arm around her and even though I felt her utter hopelessness, I simultaneously knew in my heart, *God has a baby for you.* While every couple is unique and their infertility challenges are different, I nevertheless believe God's desire is the same for all. I believe God has a baby for you.

Maeve's mother-in-law is a friend of mine, and she had called and asked if I would talk and pray with her distraught daughter-in-law. While I was eager to do so, I knew how radical it was to believe that God does the impossible. Thankfully, both the Bible and now my experience with many other seemingly impossible infertility situations had convinced me how much God wanted to cure her and give her children. Despite her hopelessness, I had hope in the God who does the impossible, and I could lovingly embrace Maeve with this same hope.

God Loves Fertility

I certainly did not always know that the theme of infertility and impossible pregnancy is woven inextricably into the central storyline of the Bible. The Bible starts with the fact that God the Father wants us, His children, to be fertile and have many children. Fertility, or fruitfulness (as the Bible calls it), is a theme that runs beautifully and wildly throughout the Bible. God loves big families. He loves multiplication. Over and over God instructs His people to be fertile and fruitful. God wants His image to be reproduced all over the earth. God made this very clear to the first couple, Adam and Eve. This is what is written in the Book of Genesis:

> *So God created human beings in His own image. In the image of God He created them; male and female He created them. Then God blessed them and said, "Be fruitful and multiply. Fill the earth and govern it" (Genesis 1:27-28; emphasis mine).*

Yes! God commands His children to be fruitful and to multiply. He wants us to be fertile and reproduce. He wants human beings who reflect His glory and likeness to cover the earth. And this includes you. God has a baby for you!

Infertility is Not God's Will

Infertility is *not* God's will for you. Even if your situation is dire and a cure seems impossible, that is no problem for God. In fact, God's triumph over infertility throughout the Bible and history give tremendous hope to any who are struggling to conceive. He offers that hope to you. His deepest desire is for you to be fertile and fruitful. He wants you to enjoy the gift of children. He wants to overcome every obstacle that stands in your way, because infertility is not God's will for you.

Worldwide Struggle with Infertility

Women all over the world and all throughout history have struggled with infertility. So what has gone wrong? This is a good question, because it can seem confusing, especially when we discover that God wants families to be fertile and multiply. Are some couples blessed while others are left out? Are some infertility cases too difficult for God to cure? Why is there so much infertility in the face of God's supposed desire for fruitfulness?

It is important to discern the root cause of all infertility in the world. Remember we saw that there is an evil being in the world called Satan, who is a liar and afflicter. The reality of Satan belongs to a bigger discussion about worldview.

Worldview is simply the way we perceive the world. However, it is complicated, because we are often unaware of how we see the world. We see things as we have grown to see them in our culture and family. In the Western world, we interpret situations rationally and scientifically. When it comes to having children, we naturally think this means a man and woman have sex at the right time and a baby will be conceived. We rarely think twice about this until something challenges our view. When it comes to infertility we look at it medically and physically: I cannot conceive because I do not ovulate or because I am too old or I have endometriosis. We see our infertile condition through a natural lens, a rational, scientific worldview.

Infertility and a Supernatural Worldview

However, I have found that a powerful tool for dealing with infertility is to recognize that it must also be approached with a supernatural, spiritual worldview. What do I mean? Infertility is one of the direct results of human beings' rebellion against God. This is part of the original curse that came as a result of Adam and Eve's sin in the Garden of Eden when Satan tempted them to disobey. You can read about this in the Bible, Genesis chapters two and three. After Eve disobeyed God, she was told:

> I will surely multiply your pain in childbearing; in pain you shall bring forth children. (Genesis 3:16).

God would send a Redeemer, Jesus, through a woman. Satan would bruise His heel (at the Cross), and as Jesus rose from the dead, He would bruise Satan's head, destroying his works. Infertility was one affliction Jesus would destroy.

This is not just referring to a painful labor and delivery, although that is true. I include infertility in this curse because it can be more painful than labor itself. The Hebrew word for pain used in this verse can also refer to sorrow, toil, and hardship.

Sin disrupted God's beautiful plan for a family. However, God had a plan to bring redemption from sin and all its horrific consequences, including infertility. God proclaimed to Satan:

> *I will put enmity between you and the woman, and between your offspring and her offspring; He shall bruise your head, and you shall bruise his heel (Genesis 3:15).*

God would send a Redeemer, Jesus, through a woman. Satan would bruise His heel (at the Cross), and as Jesus rose from the dead, He would bruise Satan's head, destroying his works. Infertility was one affliction Jesus would destroy.

Infertility Throughout the Bible

Infertility is also a major affliction Satan used to try to stop Jesus the Redeemer from coming. This is obvious in the Bible, because infertility afflicted the very women through whom the Redeemer would come. The entire Biblical story of Redemption unfolds through these infertile women. But God always did the "impossible": He cured their infertility, and blessed them with children. This miraculous story started with the mothers of the faith—Sarah, Rebekah, and Rachel, whose stories are recorded in Genesis. Each of these women was afflicted with the pain and sorrow of infertility. Then, the Biblical story of God curing infertility culminated with Elizabeth, the once infertile mother of John the Baptist, the forerunner of Jesus, our Redeemer.

God Cures the Impossible

The resounding theme in all of these stories is that God is a God of the impossible. He cures the infertile womb. Sarah and Elizabeth were old women who no longer even had their menstrual periods. Rebekah and Rachel struggled for 20 years before conceiving their first child. Ruth was childless for 10 years, widowed, and then married Boaz and gave birth to Obed, a son in the lineage of Jesus.

No matter how impossible your condition, God can and will bring a cure. He wants you to know that Jesus has shattered the curse on women and now women are free to be fruitful and multiply.

Infertility is a Curse

Infertility is a curse perpetrated by Satan on women and men, too. If we do not understand that we are no longer under that curse because of what Jesus has done, we can acquiesce to the infertility and live an empty, angry, bitter, childless existence. Jesus became a curse for us to free us from the curse. Paul, one of the writers in the New Testament, wrote:

Christ redeemed us from the curse of the law by becoming a curse for us—for it is written, "Cursed is everyone who is hanged on a tree" (Galatians 3:13).

Jesus hung on a tree, a cross. This freed us from the curse. Even if you do not comprehend this, Jesus wants you to know He is a healer. He is a healer of infertility. He is a healer of our deepest wounds. He is the Giver of Life. He wants to give you a healthy pregnancy, a baby, and the joyful blessing of family. He gave His very life so we might have an abundant life, filled with His blessings, including children.

Set Free from the Curse

We are set free from the curse of infertility and given the cure. This is such good news. The curse of pain and sorrow in childbearing is gone. Of course, giving birth is not entirely pain-free! It is called labor for a very good reason. But, the curse of infertility is gone. Jesus has set us free by His shed blood. Again, this may seem strange or confusing to you, but you can choose to simply believe. You can settle this in your heart and be ready to receive His blessing of a baby.

The letter to the Galatians is a powerful revelation of the freedom we now have in Christ. This touches every aspect of our lives now and forever:

Rejoice, O barren one who does not bear; break forth and cry aloud, you who are not in labor. For the children of the desolate one will be more than those of the one who has a husband (Galatians 4:27).

This verse has multiple meanings, but I urge you who are barren (infertile) to receive it as God's promise of children to you. You can rejoice loudly now, knowing you will have the joy of children.

I Know You Have Questions

At this point you might be asking, "But does all of this apply to me?" Or, you may be saying, "I really don't know if I understand or believe any of this," or "I am not good enough," or "I don't qualify," or maybe you're wondering, "How do I get in on this?" I am sure there are lots of questions swirling in your mind. That's okay!

You do not have to be perfect. You do not have to jump through a bunch of religious hoops. God just wants you to know He loves you with an unfailing love. As a good Father, He wants to give you good things. This includes children. He shows this over and over in the Bible stories of infertile women.

God really wants this gift of children for all and has made it possible for all to receive—if they so choose. You do not have to be perfect. You do not have to jump through a bunch of religious hoops. God just wants you to know He loves you with an unfailing love. As a good Father, He wants to give you good things. This includes children. He shows this over and over in the Bible stories of infertile women.

Nothing Is Too Difficult for God

"Is anything too difficult for Him?" These are the words spoken by an angel as a 90-year-old woman, Sarah, laughed when told she would soon conceive. Here is the conversation between Abraham, her husband, and three divine beings:

> *They said to him, "Where is Sarah your wife?" And he said, "She is in the tent." The Lord said, "I will surely return to you about this time next year, and Sarah your wife shall have a son." And Sarah was listening at the tent door behind him. Now Abraham and Sarah were old, advanced in years. The way of women had ceased to be with Sarah. So Sarah laughed to herself, saying, "After I am worn out, and my lord is old, shall I have pleasure?" The Lord said to Abraham, "Why did Sarah laugh and say, 'Shall I indeed bear a child, now that I am old?' Is anything too hard for the Lord? At the appointed time I will return to you, about this time next year, and Sarah shall have a son" (Genesis 18:9-14).*

And indeed she did! A year later Sarah was holding her firstborn son, Isaac, which is the Hebrew word for *laughter*. Nothing is too hard for our God! What better way to demonstrate this than to powerfully heal an infertile woman (couple) and bring forth the miracle of life from a dead womb? God wants you to be convinced of this and trust Him to do it for you. He wants you to rejoice, sing, and laugh. Not because it seems too crazy, but because it is so gloriously true! God has a baby for you.

More Encouraging Stories

There are several other stories of infertile women in the Old Testament that provide encouragement and reveal again how much the Father wants to heal this. Hannah, the mother of the prophet Samuel, vividly captures the desperation and pain many of us have felt as we witness those around us having baby after baby. Hannah's husband had another wife, Peninnah, as was the custom at that time. While the second wife was fertile and fruitful, Hannah suffered the devastation of a "closed womb." That was the understanding of the Jewish culture in regard to infertility. It is important to know that while a womb may be closed for a season, God's will is to fill it with children! Such is the story of Hannah who cried out in desperate, heartbreaking prayer even as the other wife taunted her, provoking her to painful jealousy:

> And her rival used to provoke her grievously to irritate her, because the LORD had closed her womb. So it went on year by year. As often as she went up to the house of the LORD, she used to provoke her. Therefore Hannah wept and would not eat. And Elkanah, her husband, said to her, "Hannah, why do you weep? And why do you not eat? And why is your heart sad? Am I not more to you than ten sons?"
>
> After they had eaten and drunk in Shiloh, Hannah rose. Now Eli the priest was sitting on the seat beside the doorpost of the temple of the LORD. She was deeply distressed and prayed to the LORD and wept bitterly. And she vowed a vow and said, "O LORD of hosts, if you will indeed look on the affliction of your servant and remember me and not forget your servant, but will give to your servant a son, then I will give him to the LORD all the days of his life, and no razor shall touch his head."
>
> As she continued praying before the LORD, Eli observed her mouth. Hannah was speaking in her heart; only her lips moved, and her voice was not heard. Therefore Eli took her to be a drunken woman. And Eli said to her, "How long will you go on being drunk? Put your wine away from you." But Hannah answered, "No, my lord, I am a woman troubled in spirit. I have drunk neither wine nor strong drink, but I have been pouring out my soul before the LORD. Do not regard your servant as a worthless woman, for all along I have been speaking out of my great anxiety and vexation." Then Eli answered, "Go in peace, and the God of Israel grant your petition that you have made to him." And she said, "Let your servant find favor in your eyes." Then the woman went her way and ate, and her face was no longer sad.

> *They rose early in the morning and worshiped before the* Lord; *then they went back to their house at Ramah. And Elkanah knew Hannah his wife, and the* Lord *remembered her. And in due time Hannah conceived and bore a son, and she called his name Samuel, for she said, "I have asked for him from the* Lord" *(1 Samuel 1:6-20).*

You can read the rest of Hannah and Samuel's fascinating story in the book of 1 Samuel. It is especially encouraging to note that not only did God open the womb of Hannah, but also generously filled it with at least six more children.

Dealing with Shame and Pressure

While women today do not deal with the taunts of a "sister wife" as Hannah did, some have endured shame and pressure and condemnation at the hands of their mothers, mothers-in-law, family members, and friends. It is important to be convinced of the Father's absolute desire to bless you with children so you will be strong when you encounter negative and cruel words from others, well-meaning as they sometimes are. Even if you do not struggle with others' harmful opinions, you might still battle jealousy and despair in regard to their pregnancies. You can choose to bless other pregnant women, rejoice with them, and let your faith in God be strengthened, as you know you could easily be next.

Ordinary Women Receive Miracles, Too

It was not just the well-known or important women in the Bible who received healing from infertility. Another fascinating story is found in the book of 2 Kings, where the prophet Elisha blessed a kind, hospitable woman with a miracle baby.

> *Later Elisha asked Gehazi, "What can we do for her?" Gehazi replied, "She doesn't have a son, and her husband is an old man." "Call her back again," Elisha told him. When the woman returned, Elisha said to her as she stood in the doorway, "Next year at this time you will be holding a son in your arms!"*
>
> *"No, my lord!" she cried. "O man of God, don't deceive me and get my hopes up like that." But sure enough, the woman soon became pregnant. And at that time the following year she had a son, just as Elisha had said (2 Kings 4:14-17).*

Many can relate to this woman's cry for the man of God to "not get her hopes up" with the promise of a miracle child. That is a very real response when you have endured disappointment after disappointment. However, please allow these stories and promises to get your hopes up and be assured that you, too, will soon be holding a child. God does not deceive you. God does not lie. God the Father wants to give you a child and exceed your every hope. In the above story, the prophet Elisha later raised this child from the dead. Our God is a miracle-working God. He is the Giver of Life. He loves to bless his people with His loving, powerful intervention.

Another encouragement in the Old Testament is the story of Samson. Samson was an influential, albeit controversial, judge in Israel. His mother had been unable to conceive. Then, God intervened:

> *There was a certain man of Zorah, of the tribe of the Danites, whose name was Manoah. And his wife was barren and had no children. And the angel of the* Lord *appeared to the woman and said to her, "Behold, you are barren and have not borne children, but you shall conceive and bear a son. Therefore be careful and drink no wine or strong drink, and eat nothing unclean, for behold, you shall conceive and bear a son. No razor shall come upon his head, for the child shall be a Nazirite to God from the womb, and he shall begin to save Israel from the hand of the Philistines."... And the woman bore a son and called his name Samson. And the young man grew, and the* Lord *blessed him (Judges 13:2-5, 24).*

Once again, an ordinary infertile woman conceived and gave birth to a son. God is so good!

While I do not fully understand this, it does appear from a number of stories in the Bible that God has specifically chosen in advance that certain children be born. God said to the prophet Jeremiah:

> *"Before I formed you in the womb I knew you, and before you were born I consecrated you; I appointed you a prophet to the nations" (Jeremiah 1:5).*

So, even before a child is conceived, he or she is present in the mind and heart of God. I do not believe that humans are preexistent (as some religious groups do), but I do think in some sense, God has babies that He wants born. This should strengthen our faith, especially if we struggle with infertility. Knowing God has a specific son or daughter for a couple causes me to hope in a way I may not have before.

Age is No Problem for God

Elizabeth was an older woman whose story of an impossible pregnancy is told in the New Testament book of Luke. She was filled with the shame that Jewish culture historically imposed on a woman who was unable to bear children. Nevertheless, it was obvious she loved God and lived righteously in spite of her deep sorrow:

> *In the days of Herod, king of Judea, there was a priest named Zechariah, of the division of Abijah. And he had a wife from the daughters of Aaron, and her name was Elizabeth. And they were both righteous before God, walking blamelessly in all the commandments and statutes of the Lord. But they had no child, because Elizabeth was barren, and both were advanced in years. Now while he was serving as priest before God when his division was on duty, according to the custom of the priesthood, he was chosen by lot to enter the temple of the Lord and burn incense. And the whole multitude of the people were praying outside at the hour of incense. And there appeared to him an angel of the Lord standing on the right side of the altar of incense. And Zechariah was troubled when he saw him, and fear fell upon him. But the angel said to him, "Do not be afraid, Zechariah, for your prayer has been heard, and your wife Elizabeth will bear you a son, and you shall call his name John. And you will have joy and gladness, and many will rejoice at his birth, for he will be great before the Lord. And he must not drink wine or strong drink, and he will be filled with the Holy Spirit, even from his mother's womb. And he will turn many of the children of Israel to the Lord their God, and he will go before him in the spirit and power of Elijah, to turn the hearts of the fathers to the children, and the disobedient to the wisdom of the just, to make ready for the Lord a people prepared" (Luke 1:5-17).*

This story is continued in Luke 1, concluding with:

> *After these days his wife Elizabeth conceived, and for five months she kept herself hidden, saying, "Thus the Lord has done for me in the days when he looked on me, to take away my reproach among people" (Luke 1:24-25).*

Later, when the angel Gabriel told Mary, the mother of Jesus, that she would become pregnant by the Holy Spirit, the angel added:

> *And behold, your relative Elizabeth in her old age has also conceived a son, and this is the sixth month with her who was called barren. For nothing will be impossible with God (Luke 1:36-37).*

He is the God of the Impossible—not one bit thwarted by old age! He is a truly loving God who delights in demonstrating that nothing is impossible with Him.

Infertile Women Have Prominent Sons

Often, the pattern in Scripture is that the child born from an infertile woman goes on to have a prominent role in God's plan. This was true of the sons of Sarah, Rebekah, Rachel, Ruth, Hannah, Manoah's wife, and Elizabeth. All had sons who went on to have significant destinies in God's plan. This does not guarantee the absence of heartache or struggle with the child. However, it does compel parents to trust the Father for His work and His destiny for their children.

I can assure you that God wants to bless you. It is important to know the truth that the Cross of Jesus made it possible for all of us to receive the tremendous blessing of the Father—including the blessing of fertility.

God Does Not Play Favorites

Although these accounts are filled with strange and miraculous events, please know that this same God is still doing miracles, and He does not play favorites, though it can seem like it at times. God wants to give you a healthy pregnancy, healthy baby, and the joyful blessing of family. He gave His very Son, Jesus, so we might have an abundant life, filled with His blessings, including children. He wants to bless you, too. God has a baby for you. Every story and every situation in the Bible and in life is unique, just as you are unique. Yet, I can assure you that God wants to bless you. It is important to know the truth that the Cross of Jesus made it possible for all of us to receive the tremendous blessing of the Father—including the blessing of fertility.

God Loves Our Dependence on Him

So much of Scripture testifies to the overwhelming grace of God in the lives of all kinds of people. God certainly does not choose perfect people for His work. On the other hand, He loves it when we recognize that apart from Him, we can do nothing. Jesus said it this way:

I am the vine; you are the branches. Whoever abides in me and I in him, he it is that bears much fruit, for apart from me you can do nothing (John 15:5).

We have the incredible privilege of living in union with God. This indwelling results in much fruit—even the fruit of children. God loves our dependence on Him. Do not try to "be strong" in your own strength. Do not think God is looking for you to be perfect. If we could, why would we need our Savior, Jesus, the strong, perfect One, to sacrifice Himself for us, and why would we need the Holy Spirit to live inside of us? When we are weak, He is strong. His grace is sufficient:

He has said to me, "My grace is sufficient for you, for power is perfected in weakness." Most gladly, therefore, I will rather boast about my weaknesses, so that the power of Christ may dwell in me. Therefore I am well content with weaknesses, with insults, with distresses, with persecutions, with difficulties, for Christ's sake; for when I am weak, then I am strong (2 Corinthians 1:9-10).

God's grace is truly amazing. His divine favor is totally sufficient against whatever stands in the way of your pregnancy. Throughout the Bible, God makes it clear that with Him, nothing is impossible.

Read to Be Encouraged

How might you be more assured of God's cure for infertility for you? One important way is to read the Bible. I am aware that some of you who are reading this book may have never read the Bible before or maybe you do not even own a Bible. You may not even know if you believe the Bible. That's okay. I want to encourage you to read some of the stories and other Bible passages I have noted. I urge you to invite the Holy Spirit to reveal the Father's heart to you as you read His Word, study the accounts of healing and infertility, and become convinced it is God's desire to give you children.

God's Word Strengthens Faith

Soon after my husband and I received the infilling of the Holy Spirit, and the Bible became so alive and so understandable, we did a serious study on healing, infertility, and prayer in the Bible. I have listed some of the important verses throughout this book and in Appendix D because I always encourage couples to learn and then soak themselves in God's truth. This strengthens faith and brings fresh assurance of God's love and His desire to bless you with children. This may be an unfamiliar exercise for you, but it is so worth the effort. God's Word strengthens faith.

Basic Skills for Reading

However, it is important to have some basic skills for reading the Bible. The Bible can be quite confusing. One of the most important skills is making sure you put on "Son glasses." What do I mean by this? Jesus is the Son of God. His work on the Cross brought us freedom and the cure for sin and sickness, and this is critical for understanding the Bible. While the entire Bible is written *for* you, not all the Bible is written *to* you. "Put on your Son glasses" is a way of saying we need to read the Bible through the lens of what Jesus has done, or else we can be confused.

For example, all the passages about God's desire for fertility and fruitfulness, His will to cure infertility and bless couples with children, are written *for* us (and many are written *to* us) and bring an important revelation of God's will that must be our foundation. Most of these are found in the Old Testament. However, some of these passages also contain conditions we have to meet before we can receive the benefits.

For example, in Deuteronomy 28, Moses detailed the blessings and curses of the Old Covenant:

> *And if you faithfully obey the voice of the* Lord *your God, being careful to do all his commandments that I command you today, the* Lord *your God will set you high above all the nations of the earth. And all these blessings shall come upon you and overtake you, if you obey the voice of the* Lord *your God. Blessed shall you be in the city, and blessed shall you be in the field. Blessed shall be the fruit of your womb and the fruit of your ground and the fruit of your cattle, the increase of your herds and the young of your flock. Blessed shall be your basket and your kneading bowl. Blessed shall you be when you come in, and blessed shall you be when you go out* (Deuteronomy 28:1-6).

If you obey all God has said, then you will be blessed. This includes a "fruitful womb" or a fertile uterus. But, it goes on to say, if you disobey, you will be cursed. These verses are written *to* the people of God living under the Old Covenant, the old way of relating to God before Jesus set us free.

These verses are not written to us, people living under the New Covenant, the new way of relating to God. They are written *for* us. They show us God's deep desire to bless His people. We still have God's promises to bless the womb, but the blessing now comes as those living under the New Covenant of grace, not under law. We need a basic understanding of the Old and New Covenants to discern which passages apply to our lives, or else we can get confused as to how we live and relate to God. With the coming of Jesus and His work on the Cross, God's grace gushed forth, and we now have a New Covenant.

A New Covenant–Jesus Makes Us Good Enough

Jesus established a New Covenant where He personally met all the conditions that God set forth for us, then sealed it with His blood. The Book of Hebrews tells us about this New Covenant:

> *But as it is, Christ has obtained a ministry that is as much more excellent than the old as the covenant He mediates is better, since it is enacted on better promises (Hebrews 8:6).*

When we surrender our lives to Jesus and become one with Him in relationship, we are in the New Covenant with Him. He sets us free from the curses and makes a way for all the blessings. He has done all the work. He has met all the conditions. We have only to receive by faith all He has done. This is far different from striving to meet the conditions or be "good enough" so God will bless us with a baby. This faith brings honor to Jesus, the Son, because we depend on His work and His grace (unmerited favor and influence) to bring a miracle into our lives.

God's Cure is Available for All

The whole story of the Bible makes it clear that God loves family and God's cure for infertility is for all who trust Him. I have counseled many couples who were bewildered by their inability to conceive in light of their perceived "good and godly behavior." As they poured out their hearts to me they often included such statements as, "But we just don't understand. We go to church; we read our Bibles, and we live good lives. Why isn't God answering our prayer?" Others who have no religious background have been confused by the complexity of Biblical commands that they think they have to obey in order to receive a child.

Jesus makes you 100 percent acceptable to God the Father and gives you access to all His provisions. This is why I can say with confidence that God has a baby for you. We do not depend on our own goodness, perfection, or ability to obey all the commands. We rest in faith in Jesus.

Jesus makes you 100 percent acceptable to God the Father and gives you access to all His provisions. This is why I can say with confidence that God has a baby for you. We do not depend on our own goodness, perfection, or ability to obey all the commands. We rest in faith in Jesus. This is the essence of praying in faith for the blessing of children that the Father has already revealed is His will. Trusting in Jesus and praying in His Name is the tremendous privilege the Father gives us now, under the New Covenant. Again, even if you do not know Jesus yet or are uncertain about the Bible, God does believe in you and wants to answer your prayer. God has a baby for you.

A Miracle for Maeve

And God had a baby for Maeve! A small prayer team gathered around Maeve as she stood at the front of the church auditorium, accompanied by her mother-in-law. Slumped shoulders and tear-filled eyes confirmed that Maeve felt hopeless. She clearly did not want to be standing here, surrounded by strangers who knew her intimate, tragic medical history. However, we warmly introduced ourselves and then invited the presence of the Holy Spirit. We gently began to pray as He led us, waiting as always for Him to show us pictures, words, or anything else from the supernatural realm. After a brief prayer, we waited for her to speak. She said she had not thought of anything.

Then one of the prayer team members said that she had seen a picture. Pictures we see "in our mind's eye" are another way the Holy Spirit speaks. We believe this is one of His gifts mentioned in the Bible in 1 Corinthians 12—the word of knowledge—where God reveals something we did not know but He knows. While the Holy Spirit usually reveals the hindrance to the couple or person who is receiving prayer, this is not always the case. Our team member saw a picture of Maeve driving a car, steering it resolutely in one direction. She asked if Maeve had any idea of what this meant.

Almost immediately, Maeve replied, "Yes, I think it shows I always want to be in control. Especially with this infertility, I have tried and tried to take control of it. I have wanted to 'drive the car,' so to speak." I then recalled a verse I had recently read in a contemporary version of the Bible, the Message. Jesus is speaking:

> *"Anyone who intends to come with me has to let me lead. You're not in the driver's seat; I am . . ." (Mark 8:34, MSG).*

Sometimes the Spirit highlights a verse from the Bible that is important in a prayer time. We asked Maeve if she was willing to repent from taking control—of being in the driver's seat—and let Jesus be in control, specifically in control of her fertility and having a baby.

She readily agreed, and offered a humble prayer to God, saying she was sorry for being in the driver's seat. She relinquished control of herself to Him. She said she now trusted Him for a baby.

This released faith in all of us. We blessed her womb and prayed what God gave us to pray. Her impossible medical diagnosis was being shattered by the power of faith-filled prayer. And, indeed, this was confirmed when just two months later we learned Maeve was pregnant—without any further medical intervention.

What joy we all had when she welcomed beautiful, healthy baby Sophie Rose into the world. Several months later, Maeve and her husband dedicated Sophie to the Lord. They stood in that exact spot at the front of the church where Jesus so powerfully cured her infertile womb and made it possible for her to be the joyful mother of children. Five years later, their family welcomed a second child with no medical help.

God Has a Baby for You

God has a baby for you. God wants to cure your infertility. He loves you and longs to fill your life with children, laughter, love, and joy. You can begin by just talking to Him and telling Him how you feel and what questions you have. Waiting month after month is so very, very hard. Try to concentrate on God's love for you, His promises and His goodness. Keep reading these chapters and the Bible, too, and you will have more and more insight and confidence in how God will handle your struggles and bless you with a baby.

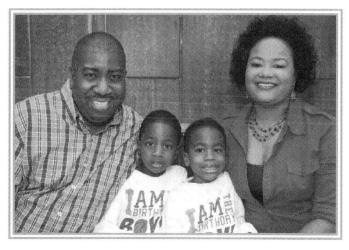

Travis, Trina, Akeel, and Amari Dixon

Important Truths for Your Journey

- Nothing is impossible with God.
- God cures infertility all throughout the Bible.
- Jesus has set you free from the curse of infertility.

Suggested Action Steps

- Begin your own Bible Study on infertility. See Appendix D for helpful resources.
- Continue to ask God questions and listen for thoughts.

Other Hindrances to Conception

"There is nothing medically wrong; we just can't conceive."

"There is absolutely nothing wrong with me or my husband!" Sandra cried, shaking her head in perplexity. Her husband Jeremy looked on helplessly and added, "We can't figure out what is stopping us from getting pregnant." They went on to explain that they had been trying for several years and were especially frustrated because the doctor assured them there was nothing physically interfering with pregnancy. They were both perfectly healthy in every way and should easily conceive. There was nothing medical science could specifically do to help.

While that should be good news to most, I have found that it can be disappointing for couples to discover there is actually nothing they can fix with drugs, surgery, or other procedures. There may be simple natural hindrances they can address with a few adjustments, or, more likely, there are spiritual hindrances that need to be exposed and removed. Many couples are unaware of these spiritual hindrances, however, and are only looking for medical or natural remedies.

Simple "Natural" Hindrances

Though the Internet is overflowing with all kinds of information to help couples conceive, I am regularly amazed at the ignorance I encounter. Sometimes the wife has limited understanding of her cycle and timing of ovulation and hence, the prime time for conceiving. The inability to conceive may simply be a matter of having sex on the wrong days. Some men are unaware of the sperm production pattern and may need to adjust frequency of sex in order to have maximum fertility. There is wisdom in being well versed in some basics of reproduction, which may eliminate natural hindrances and result in conception.

Spiritual Hindrances

However, when I discover there is no known medical issue of infertility to be cured and the couple is well informed, I know that we have most likely encountered a spiritual hindrance. We learned about this aspect in previous chapters when we saw that there is another realm, which includes supernatural influences from Satan, which can contribute to infertility.

Through interacting with hundreds of infertile couples, I have discovered there are specific spiritual hindrances when it comes to getting pregnant.

Through interacting with hundreds of infertile couples, I have discovered there are specific spiritual hindrances when it comes to getting pregnant. I will share some of these in this chapter. These hindrances are sometimes directly linked to physical problems, but not always. Since I know, and you are learning, that it is absolutely God's desire to cure infertility and bless couples with children, then we can be fairly confident there is something specifically hindering conception when couples cannot conceive even though they have been told all is well. But how do we figure out what these hindrances are and how do we remove them?

Thankfully, we have the Holy Spirit who can reveal what we need to know. He is more than willing and is even eager to expose hindrances. I know this may sound strange to some, so I will give further explanation and instruction. Then I will explain how to remove the hindrances so conception can occur.

Imperfect Past

Right away when I say spiritual hindrance, many people think I am referring to sin or ungodly behavior. They think their imperfect behavior or lifestyle or past mistakes are major hindrances to receiving from God. Others think they have to be "good enough" or somehow "qualified" in order to receive God's cure for infertility. Others are fearful that they must permanently suffer the consequences of poor choices that have resulted in STDs, abortions, or eating disorders that damaged their bodies or emotions. Does an imperfect past doom one to a childless future? No!

Sins Forgiven

I want to be very clear here. From God's side, sin does not hinder you. Jesus took away all sin. This is the amazing truth of what Jesus has done for all of us. All of our sin is removed by faith in Jesus and His work on the Cross. His blood makes us clean, blameless, and holy. All our sins are gone—past, present, and future. We are made new, and nothing stands between us and God's love and power. Even though we may at times struggle with sinful actions and attitudes, Jesus has forgiven us. In addition, Jesus also took our sicknesses and diseases, including infertility, and made it possible for us to receive healing from harmful consequences, genetic conditions, and "unknown" afflictions:

> *But he was pierced for our transgressions; he was crushed for our iniquities; upon him was the chastisement that brought us peace, and with his wounds we are healed (Isaiah 53:5).*

Sin Consciousness Can Destroy Faith

However, many of us were raised in traditions where we were especially "sin-conscious." We were always examining ourselves for sin or confessing our known sins to others—big and small. We lived in fear that if this was not done, we could be sent to hell or punished. Or in the case of infertility, we would be denied a child. This is blatantly wrong! This is false. This type of thinking obscures and diminishes the absolute glory of Jesus's sacrifice on our behalf on the cross. Sin consciousness destroys our ability to believe. All our sins have been removed, and we stand blameless and clean in our Father's sight. This is not on account of any work we have done, but all on the basis of our faith in the work Jesus has done.

Savior Conscious, Not Sin Conscious

This may seem foreign to some or unclear, but all you have to do is tell Jesus you trust Him or want to trust Him and need His help. He will actually give you a new heart, not physically, but you do become a brand new person. You now belong to Jesus Christ:

> *This means that anyone who belongs to Christ has become a new person. The old life is gone; a new life has begun And all of this is a gift from God, who brought us back to himself through Christ (2 Corinthians 5:17-18).*

This is all a gift from God. He absolutely saved us from all sin. Jesus Christ is a Savior—the one and only Savior. Let's be Savior conscious, not sin conscious. God reminds us that He does not remember our sins and bad behavior:

> *I will remember their sins and their lawless deeds no more (Hebrews 10:17).*

Jesus does not remember our sins. Jesus dealt with our sins. Why do I address this so strongly?

Infertility is Not a Punishment

I have seen infertile couple after infertile couple think their infertility is a direct punishment for their sin. No! Jesus took their punishment for sin. However, just thinking that their sin is a problem is indeed a real hindrance to faith. So, it is important during our times of counsel and prayer that we discern if such thinking is hindering them. We want to make sure people understand that sin cannot stop the blessing of God. However, if someone believes that it does, that can be a hindrance. Believing a lie can give Satan a way to hinder conception.

Satan Fills Our Minds with Lies

Of course, Satan is the major hinderer. Remember, he is a liar and is busy filling our minds with lies. Satan wants to stop fertility. We already established how much he has cursed women throughout history with infertility. He has used different obstacles to hinder the faith of struggling couples. He is the thief. He is a liar. He is clever and has many devices up his sleeve. But we do not have to be afraid or anxious. Jesus's disciple Peter instructed us about this:

> *Stay alert! Watch out for your great enemy, the devil. He prowls around like a roaring lion, looking for someone to devour. Stand firm against him, and be strong in your faith (1 Peter 5:8-9).*

We can be aware and stand firm and strong in faith—faith in our good Father who wants to bless us. This means we can keep choosing to trust God even when we may not feel like it or when our circumstances do not look good. We can trust God to show us any hindrances.

One of the main activities of the Holy Spirit is to show us truth. He can reveal what we need to know, even those things hidden deep in our subconscious. Truth brings freedom (as John 8:32 says, ". . . and you will know the truth, and the truth will set you free"). Truth strengthens faith. Truth exposes any lies we have believed.

The Holy Spirit Shows Us Truth

One of the main activities of the Holy Spirit is to show us truth. He can reveal what we need to know, even those things hidden deep in our subconscious. Truth brings freedom (as John 8:32 says, ". . . and you will know the truth, and the truth will set you free"). Truth strengthens faith. Truth exposes any lies we have believed.

So how do we receive truth from the Holy Spirit? The Holy Spirit often "pops" things into our minds. It is not a voice from the outside, just a thought we had never really had before. This is one of the most common ways God speaks. It is quite simple, and anyone can "hear."

Listening to the Holy Spirit in this way is important when we meet with couples to talk and pray. As we began to pray for Sandra and Jeremy, I invited the Holy Spirit to show them anything that was hindering their conception of a child. I explained they should not try to dredge up anything but to be aware of a thought or picture that might "pop" into their mind. I had already reminded them that infertility and conception were very spiritual issues, as shown throughout the Bible. I had illustrated a few of the "hindrance hooks," as I like to call them, that I have encountered.

Satan Uses Our Sexual Past

Because infertility has to do with reproduction, one of Satan's main tools to hinder couples is their sexual history. This may include promiscuity, abortion, or other shameful things that Satan taunts them with. However, sexual issues are not the only things in his arsenal, as I will share a bit later. I also inform the couple that the Holy Spirit is quick to respond to our request to show us hindrances. Therefore, each person should be extra alert for what "pops" in his or her mind. Share the first thought, picture, word, or memory that comes when we pray. If you start to think about this too deeply, you dredge things up that really have no relevance to the prayer time.

After I asked the Holy Spirit to reveal any hindrance, Sandra looked up rather sheepishly and said, "I have a thought that popped into my mind." She glanced at her husband as if she needed permission to share and he merely looked down. "Well," she continued, "we were high school sweethearts and devout Christians. We were both committed to wait to have sex until our wedding night. This was very important to us and to our family. However, on the night before our wedding, we gave in to our passions. We had sex. We were so ashamed. We were actually devastated. We did confess this to our pastor, but this still haunts us."

No Formulas for Prayer

I knew right away we had exposed the hindrance. Next, we waited a moment to hear how the Holy Spirit would direct us to pray. There are no formulas here. Every couple is different. Every situation is unique. The only similarity is the outcome—a healthy baby. As I waited, I had a sense of how this "night of passion" was being used by Satan to hinder their faith for a baby. I began to pray to remove all shame, guilt, and condemnation by the shed blood of Jesus. I saw how Satan convinced them they had to "pay" for their sin (how wrong, since Jesus did this at a great cost—His own life). I then spoke directly to them as a couple, saying Jesus saw them as worthy of becoming parents. Jesus saw them as whole, clean, and holy—cleansed by His blood and made new by His work.

Next, I asked Sandra and Jeremy to repent—turn from—the lies of Satan that were keeping them in bondage and shame. They were still thinking that their sinful action prevented them from becoming parents. They saw themselves as unworthy to receive God's blessings. They were trying to atone for their sin. I asked them to verbalize their faith in Jesus's blood that had already cleansed them and made them worthy. Then the team prayed over them, blessing their bodies to release the healthy egg and sperm to be united as the child the Father was so longing to give them.

Freedom Comes!

There were many tears. Freedom had come. All of us could feel it. Hindrances to faith had been removed. We had discovered "the hook" with the Holy Spirit's help. We were all confident that good news would follow soon. Thus, a short four weeks later, I was not surprised to learn that Sandra was pregnant. I was of course overjoyed once again at the greatness of our God. I was reassured of His deep desire to bless His children with children. Sandra and Jeremy are now the parents of three rambunctious sons. Nothing could ultimately stand in the way of God's cure for their infertility.

Not every counsel and prayer session results in such a quick conception. However, time after time I have witnessed the Holy Spirit reveal "the hindrance hook" that has hindered a couples' faith, and I knew they would conceive in the fullness of time.

Oh, how Satan distorts the glorious Gospel of Jesus Christ! How he twists the true meaning of the Cross. Thankfully, the Holy Spirit reveals the truth that sets people free—free to conceive and give birth to the child God wants to give them.

Secret Sin

I do want to make sure you understand one thing about the issue of sin, though. Sometimes, there is a "secret sin" that one or both of the couple are still committing when they come for prayer. This is a different situation than when you are dealing with sin that has been confessed, repented of, and is no longer an active issue in your life, but the shame is hindering your faith. As in Sandra and Jeremy's situation, I reassure couples that the blood of Jesus has taken sin away completely. I remind them that only their unbelief hinders them from living in the reality of the forgiveness and freedom that is already theirs.

However, there are some who may not be walking in the truth of this and may still be in bondage to sin. There may be the presence of what I call "secret sin" or immoral behavior going on, perhaps without the other spouse knowing. This can be a serious hindrance.

The Holy Spirit Reveals

The Holy Spirit is faithful to reveal this hindrance—not with condemnation, but with the hope that freedom and forgiveness is already theirs, waiting to be received by faith.

One couple, Ted and Joy, revealed that when we prayed for the Spirit to show the "hindrance hook," they both were convicted about watching pornographic movies together. They had started to do this to enhance their sexual encounters that had become wearisome and difficult through their struggle with infertility.

This weariness is often the case when a couple gets so burdened with timed sex, repeated sex, and the spontaneity and excitement have worn thin. The watching of these movies was something the Spirit brought to both of their minds as an unhealthy activity.

Again, while the blood of Jesus has already taken this sin away and the Father has forgiven them and forgotten this sin, Satan was keeping them in bondage to a sinful practice. They were filled with shame and condemnation, knowing this was not God's best for their sexual intimacy. Their faith in God's power and love was hindered. The repentance (turning from) this activity actually brought so much healing to their marriage. In addition, they have fresh faith in God's desire to give them a child. They are learning to enjoy sexual intimacy again. They are resting in God's love and assurance that they will soon be announcing the good news of "We're pregnant!"

Hiding the Truth

Paul and Suzanne had already suffered through two miscarriages. They were young and healthy. The doctors could give no medical reason for her failure to carry a baby past nine weeks. Being a nurse, she was quite familiar with all the medical infertility research and options. At this point, they both knew they needed God's help. Our team waited for the Holy Spirit to speak to them. Suzanne shared several things, but Paul was unusually silent. We proceeded with prayer, but I knew in my heart that we had not discerned the true hindrance. However, we do not force couples to come up with something. If they do not have a sense and our team is not getting anything definite, then we bless them. We ask Jesus for healing and the gift of a child. And this is what we did.

Months passed and I never heard any news from them. Then one day, a friend shared that Paul had confessed to an extramarital affair and he and Suzanne were now getting marriage counseling in hopes of saving their marriage. While I was distraught by this revelation, I now knew why our prayer time had been less than effective: Paul had not been willing to confess his ongoing sinful activity. He was hiding the truth. And, of course, it was a sin that was directly related to conception. He was having sex with a woman who was not his wife. This is very serious. Sin is real. Sin is destructive. Their marriage was not healthy. It would have been damaging to bring a newborn into that hostile environment. I am so thankful God did not answer our prayer for a child when we first prayed for them.

Healed Marriage, Healed Bodies

About a year and a half later, I had the opportunity to pray with them again. They were holding hands and beamed with love. Their marriage had been miraculously restored. This is no light thing. Adultery crushes a marriage. The wounding from unfaithfulness is deep and gaping. It takes God's abundant grace and His gift of forgiveness to bring healing. It takes God's love and strength to restore shattered trust.

May I just pause here and say this is a word of encouragement for some of you? Perhaps adultery has shattered your marriage. You are still together, but right now you are thinking that a child will save your marriage. No! A thousand times no! Please get God's help—through your church or a seasoned counselor.

Thankfully, Paul and Suzanne had received God's gracious redemption. They had made a fresh start. They were ready to receive the gift of a healthy pregnancy and child. God was ready to bless them. We prayed a simple prayer, just three short minutes, asking God to give them a child. Ten months later, Suzanne gave birth to an adorable daughter, Gracie Lee. Together they gave heartfelt thanks to God for His indescribable goodness.

Each Hindrance is Unique

I hesitate to give too many examples of the "hindrance hooks," because I don't want you to try to figure this out for yourselves based on others' stories. I am confident the Holy Spirit will show each couple what is presently hindering pregnancy in their lives. However, I will share several more examples to encourage your faith that the Spirit so longs to reveal anything that hinders your faith in Jesus for a child.

> Every couple has struggles—whether it is infertility or infidelity or just the inability to get along. It never does any good to compare to others. God wants to bring His full redemption to every person's life no matter how the enemy or our own selfishness has brought ruin or disappointment.

Remember, every couple is unique, and the hindrances are specific to each couple. I know it can seem unfair, too, that you actually have hindrances when so many other couples get pregnant just looking at each other. Others' lives are a total wreck, filled with sin, troubles, and all kinds of ungodly stuff, and yet they have no trouble conceiving. Please do not go there. That is not helpful. Every couple has struggles—whether it is infertility or infidelity or just the inability to get along. It never does any good to compare to others. God wants to bring His full redemption to every person's life no matter how the enemy or our own selfishness has brought ruin or disappointment. He knows exactly how to bless you!

Jealousy Can Hinder

Anna had suffered multiple miscarriages during her five-year marriage to Liam. When we met to pray, we first took authority over a spirit of death. This means I used the Holy Spirit's power in me to release Anna from any possible oppression by simply saying, "Any spirit of death that remains in this womb must go in Jesus's name." I always do this if miscarriage—death of a baby—has occurred. I want to make sure the womb is cleansed from any oppressing spirits. This may seem odd or weird, but when you embrace a supernatural worldview, you have clearer understanding.

Then we waited to see what the Holy Spirit would reveal to Anna and Liam as a possible hindrance to their faith. Sure enough, a thought popped in her head. "Well," she said, "I really don't know if this is important, but I keep thinking how angry and jealous I have been that my sister has had no trouble getting pregnant, and I have struggled so much. Every time she announces another pregnancy, I can barely stand to be around her. I know I should be happy for her, but I am so angry and so jealous."

I knew this was the Spirit. This is actually a fairly common hindrance for women. When jealousy is a problem, it means that you have not settled in your heart that God wants to give you a baby, too. You may think you are being overlooked, and you are angry. Of course, you may not verbalize it this way. But the jealousy you are feeling is a telling symptom of a deeper problem in your heart. You are not convinced it is God's absolute desire to bless you with a baby.

I have known infertile women who refused to go to baby showers, even of very close friends, because their jealousy, anger, and depression were too overwhelming.

When I heard what Anna said, I invited the Holy Spirit to come and reveal to her and Liam that it is indeed God's will to bless them with a baby. I then instructed them to let that sink in and be ready to repent from believing that God was not going to bless them, too. I waited until they were able to say a brief prayer telling God they were sorry for not believing this, asking Him to fill their hearts with His truth and His faith.

I am always amazed at how the Spirit moves to convince people of the Father's love for them and His desire to bless them with a child—especially after they allow the Spirit to remove that hindrance of doubt that the jealous anger indicated was there.

This newfound faith will probably be tested when another person announces her pregnancy. But even if jealousy tries to rear its ugly head again, you can simply refuse to allow it to surface, reminding yourself of the Father's love and His desire and faithfulness to give you a child. Thank Him for His gift. Rejoice with the new parents. Host the next baby shower. You know your baby shower is coming soon.

Offer to pray for another couple that is struggling to conceive. Give away the faith in your heart and watch the Father pour more into yours. No more jealousy. Just a joyful waiting for what you know is yours.

Anna and Liam went away rejoicing. They were free from the hindrance of jealousy. They believed God wanted to bless them. They thanked Him for His love. And, yes, it was not long before Anna became pregnant, carried her baby full term, and they became the proud parents of a feisty daughter, Olivia Mae. They eventually welcomed three more daughters into their happy home. The hindrance of jealousy was gone, and joy flooded their lives.

Control Can Hinder

Control can be a powerful hindrance when it comes to conception. Control is a big issue in our lives. We want control—control of our emotions, bodies, families, money, lives—and so much more! However, when we become children of God, we make the decision to surrender that control to our loving Father. We are no longer in control. Jesus is our Lord. He is a wonderful boss. He really does know what is best for us at all times. However, in the course of our lives, when things are not going fast enough or in the way we want, we can easily think we know better. We want things to go our way. We try to take control. Control is a big issue that I have seen hinder faith over and over. It is different in each person's life. But the Holy Spirit is faithful to show how it is a hindrance to faith for fertility.

Allie had been trying to get pregnant for about five years when she came for prayer. Control was an issue in her life, too, but in a different manner than it had been for Maeve. Again, every person is unique. While the hindrance may be the same—shame, control, jealousy, anger—the way it manifests in one's life differs from person to person.

When we asked the Spirit to show Allie what the hindrance was to her faith, she recalled making a very interesting vow. Allie had been mercilessly teased and tormented by her brothers while they were growing up. Because of this, she had made the statement, "'When I am a mother, I will NEVER have a baby boy!" She realized she had tried to take control of what gender her baby would be. She wanted God to have that control. She had never actually connected her vow with her inability to fully trust Jesus for a baby. She had basically forgotten she had even ever uttered that vow.

But now, she received the Father's forgiveness for taking control by speaking the vow. She said she would trust God for the gift of a child, boy or girl. With the authority of Jesus's name, we broke the power of that vow and Satan's use of it to stop the conception of a child. We blessed her womb to be filled with a boy or girl, as the Father willed. One year later, she and her husband joyfully welcomed baby Joseph Andrew, their firstborn child, and their firstborn son. The hindrance of control had been hammered.

> I have literally hundreds of stories where hindrances were revealed, removed, and couples conceived. Every couple and every situation is different. Sometimes there is a combination of natural, medical, and spiritual issues. Sometimes it's just spiritual hindrances. No matter, God wants to show you anything that stands in the way of you having a baby.

God Will Show You

I have literally hundreds of stories where hindrances were revealed, removed, and couples conceived. Every couple and every situation is different. Sometimes there is a combination of natural, medical, and spiritual issues. Sometimes it's just spiritual hindrances. No matter, God wants to show you anything that stands in the way of you having a baby. Don't be discouraged by those who seem unhindered in their ability to conceive. Be encouraged that God wants to show you.

Ask God to reveal to you what is hindering your conception of the child He longs to give you. Remember, He is ready to tell you. This is not waiting for some audible voice from Heaven or some vivid dream in the night, although God can speak in those ways, too. Usually, this is simply listening to ideas or images that "pop" into your head, and then sharing with your spouse so you can pray together.

Again, do not try to think too deeply or too long about this. Say, "Holy Spirit, please show us what is hindering our conception." Then be still and wait for a picture, a word, a thought, or just a sense. It may not come right away, but you will discover later that day or even that week that you suddenly are aware of an incident or scenario that came to you "out of the blue," and you will want to pray about it.

I am keenly aware of how much God wants your child to be born. He loves you. He loves your unborn child. He is eager to reveal and remove any hindrance to this reality in your life. Ask Him!

Jenny and Eric's Story

I want to conclude this chapter with the story of Jenny and Eric Shanley. This young couple from New Hampshire wrote out the details of their journey through infertility. I think their story so captures many of the important elements I have discussed so far. I have taken the liberty, with their permission, to arrange what they wrote into story form. Enjoy and be encouraged!

> *We were so eager to start a family, and like most couples, we thought it would be easy. After trying for a year with no success, we knew something was wrong. We had a series of tests, and our subsequent treatment was laparoscopic surgery to remove a polyp in my (Jenny's) fallopian tube. In addition, I was diagnosed with PCOS (polycystic ovary syndrome), and took Metformin and adjusted my diet to treat that. We went on to struggle for six years, from 2004 to 2010. After following all the medical procedures and recommendations, we learned that the doctor we were seeing (the only one in our area) was closing his practice in 2009. He said there was really nothing else he could do for us. At this point, he saw no reason for any issues with conception (other than what we already knew), and that there was no need for further treatment. However, there was no pregnancy!*
>
> ### Doubting God
>
> **Even though we are committed Christians, throughout this** *journey we oscillated in our confidence that we would actually have children. At times, we were so sure God would bless us, and then there were times when we doubted and weren't so sure. These times of doubt brought on feelings of anger and serious depression. I (Jenny) found myself questioning God's goodness. I've always said, "God does whatever He wants"—referring to God's sovereignty. I knew that it was no big thing for a powerful, sovereign God to do this, and yet He was allowing us to go through this painful season in our lives.*

This was confusing to me and hindered my faith. We of course received prayer from people in our church family. We shared our fears, bitterness, discouragement, and dashed dreams with others who listened patiently and loved us. Yet it was so frustrating seeing other couples get pregnant without having any challenges. I kept wondering why God would allow others who didn't even want children to get pregnant. He knew we felt like we were ready and willing to have children and love them very much!

Frustrations!

It was really frustrating when people gave us medical advice and recommendations on "how to get pregnant"! But one of the most impacting moments for me (Eric) was when one of our church members came up to me and just plainly said, "I'm so sorry you are going through this. We love you both so much."

We were both just about to quit and give up. We had succumbed to the "fact" that it was just the way it was. There was the real possibility that we would never conceive, never have children of our own. We had pretty much settled that "reality" in our hearts. We did not realize how wrong this belief actually was. The Holy Spirit showed me (Jenny) that I was gripped by my own fear of not knowing what was going to happen. This was directly keeping me from allowing the Lord to do what He had wanted to do for me! God wanted me to know that it is His will for us to conceive and to have children of our own! I was about to learn this in a powerful way.

God Speaks

It was the summer of 2010, and we were attending The Vineyard Church Summer Regional Conference in the Poconos of Pennsylvania. The first night, Phil Strout (our national director) spoke about being "all in." This was a divine moment for me in my relationship with God. I decided that I was going to give Him control, and throw it all in! At that point, I thought that meant that He didn't want me to have children, and I was willing to give that up to Him, even though I was very angry and upset with Him about this.

So, the next morning, Dianne Leman was speaking. Her message wasn't directly related to our story, but she did share her background/story about their struggles with infertility and how God brought them through that season. I don't honestly remember much of what she said, except this: "The truth is, God wants you to have children!" This renewed my hope. So she then concluded, and as with any Vineyard conference, there was ministry time at the end.

Receiving Prayer

My father noticed that Dianne was praying for women who were having trouble with conceiving and having children. I went over to receive prayer. When she started praying for me, she told me that oftentimes when women have issues getting pregnant, they can have a "hook," something keeping them from getting pregnant, and that God was after something. So she began praying that God would show me what that "hook" was in my life. She got a word of knowledge from the Holy Spirit that I had let my fears and uncertainty get in the way of God doing what He wanted to do in my life. We prayed together, and I asked for forgiveness in trying to take and keep control of my own life!

Renewed Hope and Faith

Leaving the conference left us with a renewed hope and faith for what God was going to do. Several weeks after the conference, we decided to be intentional about preparing our life for a future with children. We would act on our newfound faith. I gave my six-week notice at my job (where I had been a nanny for a family for the past three years). I let them know that I needed to have time to prepare for a family of my own.

Pregnant!

I didn't know it at the time, but I actually got pregnant before my six weeks was up! In taking this step of faith, I had an awesome pregnancy where I was able to relax and get the rest that I needed in preparing for our first child. God is so good! Emmaline Jean was born on 6/18/2011. She truly is our miracle baby. But, God is a God of abundance! In 2013, I got pregnant again, and Elias Timothy was born on 4/7/2014. He is beyond amazing!

God Loves You!

For those of you who are waiting for God to bless you with a baby . . . Know that God doesn't need any reason to show us His love, as He already did that at the Cross. But He shows us His love in this area, because of His love! Know, too, that God truly is for you, and that His promises are sure. Allow God to go deep during this time of waiting—the thing that's keeping you from getting pregnant may not be a physical matter at the core. He will be faithful to show you what is hindering you, and He will do the impossible for you! Trust Him!

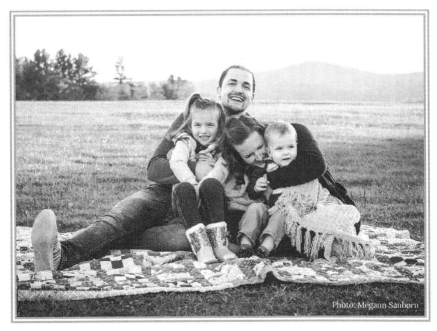

Eric, Jenny, Emma and Eli Shanley

A Thank You

Jenny sent me this accompanying note to her story:

> Hey Dianne,
>
> Thank you for thinking of me and giving me a chance to put our story out there to help others the way that you helped me. We had a young couple come to our church last week, and she had shared with a small group how she had been pregnant and ended up losing her baby. Most of the people in our church know the struggle that Eric and I went through to get pregnant, so on Sunday my Dad asked me to pray for her. He said that because it was something I had received healing for, that he felt I was the right person to pray for her in the same way. Even though it has been four years since the day I received healing, it had never occurred to me that what I received was not just for *me*. And I realized that I now have something more to give, because God very rarely gives us something just for us to keep, but so that it can flow out of us and be given to other people.

So, thank you for sharing your gift with me. It has changed my life in ways that I see every day when I look at my two beautiful children. And thank you for giving me one more place to pass on the gift that I received, by sharing our story. I know that many more lives will be healed and changed through this book and I can't wait to see the fruit of it!

Thank you again!

Love, Jenny

Your Story

You will have a wonderful story to share. You, like Jenny and Eric, will have new prayers to pray for others as you give away what God has so freely given to you. Let the Holy Spirit reveal any hindrances that Satan has put in the way of your miracle.

The next section unfolds how to receive God's cure for your infertility. You will learn how to ask God, believe God, and cooperate with each other and with God on your way to receiving God's gift of a child.

Important Truths for Your Journey

- There may be both physical and spiritual hindrances to your fertility.
- Satan focuses on lies about God and our situations; the Spirit reveals truth.
- Every couple is unique, and what is a hindrance to one is not to another.
- God will be faithful to show you what hinders you.

Suggested Action Steps

- Ask the Holy Spirit to show you your hindrance. Be alert for what pops up in your mind, and share it with your spouse.
- Read the next section for specific instructions on what to do with what the Holy Spirit reveals to you.

PART III

Receiving God's Gift of Fertility

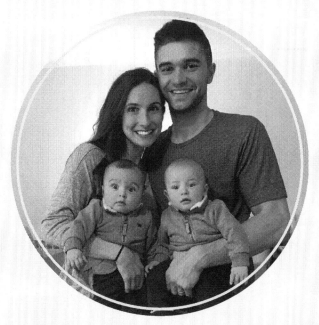

Teresa and Trent Meacham welcomed twins Andrew and Malachi

Addressing dilemmas and reading others' stories can help bring hope to your hearts, but you still need specific directions on what you can actually do to receive God's cure for infertility for you. These chapters will give you clear instructions on how to pray, how to trust God, and how to cooperate with His help so you can receive God's gift of fertility and His gift of a child.

Praying with Boldness and Confidence

"We don't know how to pray!"

Julie and her husband Mike had thoroughly enjoyed their first few years of married life without children. In addition to travel, friends, dining out, and a new home purchase, Julie was a busy reading teacher at the local middle school. Mike was pursuing a challenging career in the biotech field. They, like most young couples, were confident they could start a family when they wanted.

"Getting pregnant is easy—right? Let's wait until we are ready." That was their thinking, and maybe some of you can identify with it. So many young couples are waiting to start their families. Demanding careers and mountainous college debt are obvious and sensible reasons to delay. Exciting, accessible travel and the ease of birth control contribute to the enjoyment of an extended childless marriage. Many couples want to purchase their first home and get settled before having children. Most think getting pregnant will be easy and they will abandon contraception when they are ready.

Not So Easy

Well into Mike and Julie's deliberate attempts to conceive, Julie knew something was not right. She was not pregnant after almost a year of unprotected sex. And now, her menstrual cycle seemed to have come to a crashing halt. Frantic searches on the plethora of infertility websites only served to throw her into a more desperate emotional state. Something was wrong. This was not easy!

No Formulas

She came to me, her mother, to ask for prayer. She was not sure how to ask God, how to pray. She needed a cure for her possible infertility, and of course knew my experience and my confidence in God. As I held my distraught daughter, how I wished I had a formula to quickly correct her problem and pronounce her cured. But I knew I didn't have any such formula. Faith and friendship is God's way, not formulas. I did have that strong belief in God's desire to give her a child (my grandchild, no less!), and I knew He would show her and Mike how to ask, believe, and cooperate with Him. But there was no quick and easy formula. Receiving God's cure for infertility is simple, but not necessarily easy.

Three Simple Actions

Even though I have divided this section into three parts, I want to be clear that there is no set formula for receiving God's cure for infertility. These chapters discuss three simple actions that all can do. Every couple can ask, believe, and cooperate—three actions that are as simple as ABC. But, every couple and every situation is different, so some steps will be easier or harder, depending on the couple. Some will find one aspect easy but struggle with another. In spite of the differences, one thing is the same: God desires to cure you of infertility and give you a child. God loves you and wants to relate to you as you learn to receive His cure for your infertility.

Prayer = Asking

The most popular word for prayer in the Bible is the word "ask." Over and over we are invited to talk with God, our Father, about our needs and desires and ask Him for His help. But prayer can be a confusing topic. Some of you may have never prayed. Others have never prayed out loud or have only whispered words from a Book of Common Prayer. Many do not realize that prayer is simply talking with God, and that includes asking Him for what we need and desire.

Ask God the Father with Confidence

It is so wonderful that we can simply ask God for what we want, and we can do this with confidence in our hearts and receive the help we need. We can draw near to His throne—another way to describe His Presence—and ask Him for help:

> *Let us then with confidence draw near to the throne of grace, that we may receive mercy and find grace to help in time of need (Hebrews 4:16).*

Our Father is a good Father! He wants to give us good gifts. What better invitation do we need than to approach Him in prayer and ask Him for help? We can learn to pray with boldness and confidence.

Praying can be done as a couple or together with some friends. We often pray for couples with a small group of women and men, and we call this Team Prayer. I will explain that later in this chapter. First, though, I want to assure you that you can ask God for His cure and your child, and you can do this with confidence and boldness, because you are sure He hears you and wants to grant your request.

Does God Really Hear? Yes!

I have heard many people exclaim, "We have asked many times. We have prayed every possible prayer we know how to pray! We have asked in every way possible. Loud prayers. Soft prayers. Bold prayers. Timid prayers. Begging prayers. Relinquishing prayers. Others have prayed for us, too. We have asked! But, we are still waiting to be pregnant. We are really struggling. Is there a special way to ask? Does God really hear our prayer?"

What a refreshing, life-changing revelation to know that yes, God hears our prayers!

Maybe you, too, have said plenty of prayers in your life but were not sure if God heard them. Many of us grew up with rote recitations of "Now I lay me down to sleep . . ." or "God is great, God is good, Let us thank him for this food." In college, I often asked, "Help me pass this test. Get me out of this mess!" I did not really expect God to hear.

For those of you with a Catholic background, you may identify more with saying the "Our Father" or a rosary-based prayer. If by chance a prayer was answered, you may have thought it was totally random. What a refreshing, life-changing revelation to know that yes, God hears our prayers! Yes, God answers our prayers. He does have instructions for us, though.

No Repetitious Begging

While there is no special way to ask, there are some important things to know, because not every prayer is answered. Jesus is clear there is a wrong way to ask or to pray:

> *"And when you pray, do not heap up empty phrases as the Gentiles do, for they think that they will be heard for their many words. Do not be like them, for your Father knows what you need before you ask him" (Matthew 6:7-8).*

Repeated prayer is not necessary. This is how unbelievers pray. We are not unbelievers. God is our Father. He does not want His children begging. No parent enjoys that! Our Father knows our needs even before we ask, but He wants us to ask Him, showing our dependence on and love for Him. Even though He knows our needs, He often wants to talk with us about those needs and give us His wisdom.

Prayer is a Conversation

Prayer is a very relational conversation between God and you. Prayer is not a rote exercise of "getting my prayers done." No! Prayer is a rich and precious part of our relationship with the Living God. While praying, I am listening to Him. He is listening to me. I pour out my heart to Him. He assures me of His love. I ask for what I need, even though He knows. He loves my dependence on Him. He wants to show me any hindrances to conception. He is pleased by my trust in His goodness.

Prayer is a wonderful conversation. You can just begin to talk with God! Again, repeated begging is not a healthy conversation. You can ask questions about why things aren't happening or ask for help in believing when doubts come. You can ask for practical insight or just pour out your heart when you have had a difficult day. God hears you, and He especially delights in your gratitude and childlike trust.

The Prayer of Faith

God really does want to answer prayer. But He does not answer just any prayer. He answers the prayer of faith. Jesus taught this:

"And whatever you ask in prayer, you will receive, if you have faith" (Matthew 21:22).

You may be thinking, "I definitely want to receive, so how do I know if I have faith?"

God is ready to teach you how to have faith. This is just simple trust in God's goodness and love for you. Asking in faith is not some super spiritual prayer. It is asking God for what you need, assured of His love and care for you. In the next chapter I will share how to strengthen your faith, but for now, just ask with simple trust in our good God. You will not always feel like you trust Him. That is not a lack of faith. You may even be asking, "How much faith is 'enough'?" This is not an exchange game where you are trying to feel enough faith in order to get your answer. You are learning to simply believe who God is and what He says.

God Answers Specific Requests

God wants you to be specific when you ask. God delights in your faith in Him as a good Father who gives good gifts to His children. Jesus taught us how to ask:

Ask, and it will be given to you; seek, and you will find; knock, and it will be opened to you. For everyone who asks, receives, and he who seeks finds, and to him who knocks it will be opened. Or what man is there among you who, when his son asks for a loaf, will give him a stone? Or if he asks for a fish, he will not give him a snake, will he? If you then, being evil, know how to give good gifts to your children, how much more will your Father who is in heaven give what is good to those who ask Him! (Matthew 7:7-11).

Isn't this an amazing invitation and promise? And it is true. The Father wants you to ask for specific gifts.

The Father Wants to Give Us Good Gifts

He wants to give you good things, just like human parents want to give good gifts to their children. I have often had to assure people that God is not going to give them a poor substitute or an inferior answer to their prayer. When you ask God for a cure for your infertility and the gift of a child, He will not give you a substitute. He delights more in giving you good gifts than humans do in giving their very own children the good things they ask for.

Powerful Invitations to Ask

The Bible writers, speaking for God, of course, encourage us to ask. Jesus's closest friend, John, wrote one of the most powerful prayer passages:

> *Now this is the confidence that we have in Him, that if we ask anything according to His will, He hears us. And if we know that He hears us, whatever we ask, we know that we have the petitions that we have asked of Him (1 John 5:14-15).*

This was a very important verse for my husband and me when we sat down to actually write out our prayer, asking God for His cure and the gift of a child. We knew His will was to cure us and give us a baby. We had confidence that we were asking according to His will.

We Can Know God's Will

It is obviously important to know God's will. As John says . . . *if we ask anything according to His will, He hears us.* When I was first learning this amazing truth about simply asking God the Father for what I wanted, a "more spiritual" person cautioned me that this was not a carte blanche invitation to get whatever I wanted. I needed to be very sure that I was asking according to God's will. Then and only then would my prayers be answered. I found this to be a very prevalent sentiment when my husband and I visited various churches in our city that we knew believed in healing. When we asked for prayer for our infertility, they always responded, "Yes, we will pray. But we must add, 'if it be Your will, God.' That is most important."

Yes, that had been my quest, but now I had discovered what God wanted. To be honest, there were still moments when I still struggled with the question, "Is it God's will to cure ALL women of infertility?" I trusted the Holy Spirit to truly confirm this to me. I knew His desire was to bless us with children. His Word had clearly said it and His Spirit had truly anchored this in my heart. I had read and reread the stories of women who had been healed of infertility. I had written out the Bible verses that promised the gift of children. Yes, I did know without a doubt that God wanted to cure our infertility. I knew God's will was to bless us with a child.

No Presumption, Just Pleasing God

When I shared this boldly and probably too brashly with those praying for us, they quickly and authoritatively said, "Oh, you cannot be that presumptuous to expect

God to give you a child!" I never want to be presumptuous in my relationship with my Father and my prayers to Him. I want to honor His will and submit to His will at all times. But He reveals His will in so many areas through His Word and by His Spirit. This is what releases faith in our hearts so we can ask, trusting Him to give us the good things He has promised. He is so pleased by our faith in Him.

You can ask Him to cure you of infertility and give you a child. This is not a prayer of presumption. This is not a prayer of demand. This is a prayer of love for and faith in our good Father who loves to answer our prayers.

It might sound humble to say "if it be Your will" or "whatever You want, God," but when we already know His will, that is false humility. As you read the Bible verses and soak in the examples of God's cure and desire to bless you with children, you will be assured of His will. (Many of these verses are listed in Appendix D.)

You can ask Him to cure you of infertility and give you a child. This is not a prayer of presumption. This is not a prayer of demand. This is a prayer of love for and faith in our good Father who loves to answer our prayers, who loves to give us a child. And, I believe, He has actually put the desire for a child in our hearts. This is His will, not just our "selfish" desire.

Know That He Hears Us

Remember, John says:

> And if we know that He hears us, whatever we ask, we know that we have the petitions that we have asked of Him (1 John 5:15).

Do we know that he hears us? Do we have confidence that our prayers are more than words that disappear into thin air? This is very important. We want to be assured that God actually hears us and is not turning His face from us when we ask. For years, I never really knew if God heard my prayers or not. My prayers were dry recitations done out of duty and not out of a loving relationship of faith. I definitely was not confident of His unfailing love for me. I thought my bad behavior or sins of any kind prevented Him from hearing me. How wrong I was. God did hear me. The shed blood of Jesus took my sin away. Sin does not stand in the way of God hearing us and answering our prayer.

The Prerequisite is Our Faith, Not Our Perfection

We do not trust in our own ability to be perfect. Of course we want to keep our consciences clean before our Father. We love Him. We long to please Him in every way. But this is not a prerequisite for Him hearing us or answering our prayer. The "prerequisite" is our confidence, our bold faith in Him. Our confidence (faith) can grow in regards to knowing His will. We can believe what His Word says about His cure for infertility and His desire to give us children. When we sense we have confidence that God wants this for us and we know He hears us, we are ready to ask!

But first, don't forget to ask if there is any hindrance, as we discussed in Chapter 5.

Ask God to Show You Any Hindrance

Review the discussion on the types of hindrances and begin to ask the Spirit to show you if there are any hindrances blocking God's cure for your infertility. If an idea, thought, memory, or picture "pops" in your mind, consider why this might be a hindrance. Often it is a situation that Satan, the father of lies, is using to hinder your faith in God's desire to give you a child. When you recognize the lie, you can renounce it—decide to not believe it—and ask God for His truth. This usually precedes specifically asking God for your child, but not necessarily.

Ask Out Loud and in Writing

When you are ready to ask for God's cure and your child, I think it is helpful to ask God out loud and to also put your prayer in writing. We wrote out our entire prayer along with supporting Bible verses about healing, infertility, and the goodness of God. It is so easy to forget what we actually prayed.

Writing out your prayer, along with the verses from the Bible that confirm God's will, is a great reminder when you are waiting and are tempted to be discouraged. Remember, we are not repeating our request; we are just reminding ourselves and thanking God that He has heard us and is giving us our desire of a child. You can glance at it every day to affirm what you know the Father is giving to you. This also makes it easier for both husband and wife to agree wholeheartedly. I give a sample prayer in Appendix C if you need help. So, consider writing out your prayer to keep you both focused and thankful.

Pray with Others

While couples do pray together for their much-desired conception, it is also often helpful for the couple to invite a team to pray with them. This may be an unfamiliar practice for some of you, depending on your religious background. It is not an absolute by any means, but I have found team prayer to be so powerful. As you have noticed throughout these chapters, I have a strong emphasis on praying with a team of people. You may want to consider praying with friends, family, or trusted pastors. It is not necessary for these people to be ordained ministers or specially trained. However, it is wise to choose both men and women who are in agreement with the belief that God wants to cure infertility and bless couples with children. When we agree, the Father answers. Jesus modeled and taught this:

> *Again I say to you, if two of you agree on earth about anything they ask, it will be done for them by my Father in heaven (Matthew 18:19).*

So, gather those who agree with you and with God. If these people also had their own experience with God curing them of infertility or another condition, they make very good team members. They already have a vibrant faith in God's desire to cure.

Team Member Attributes

It is best if some team members are familiar with the gifts of the Holy Spirit, as these are quite helpful for prayer. The Apostle Paul talks about these gifts in 1 Corinthians:

> *A spiritual gift is given to each of us so we can help each other. To one person the Spirit gives the ability to give wise advice; to another the same Spirit gives a message of special knowledge. The same Spirit gives great faith to another, and to someone else the one Spirit gives the gift of healing. He gives one person the power to perform miracles, and another the ability to prophesy. He gives someone else the ability to discern whether a message is from the Spirit of God or from another spirit. Still another person is given the ability to speak in unknown languages, while another is given the ability to interpret what is being said. It is the one and only Spirit who distributes all these gifts. He alone decides which gift each person should have (1 Corinthians 12:7-11).*

All people can receive these gifts to give away to the couple. If you are unfamiliar with these, you can read more about them in several books listed in Appendix D.

Again, I emphasize that team members do not have to be priests or seminary-trained professionals. The most important attributes are a childlike faith in God, a love and compassion for others, a discerning spirit, and patience.

There is no infertility prayer formula. Every couple is different. Every prayer time is special. I love this. God adores each couple. He is eager to deal with their personal issues in a loving, powerful way.

How to Pray as a Team

Once again, I stress that there is no infertility prayer formula. Every couple is different. Every prayer time is special. I love this. God adores each couple. He is eager to deal with their personal issues in a loving, powerful way. However, there are some prayer-time similarities. In our groups, we set aside an hour to meet with the infertile woman or couple. While we have prayed in less time, we usually need an hour to zero in on the unique situation of each couple. If possible, we want both husband and wife to be present. Their agreement concerning the desire for a child and willingness to seek God infuses our prayer time with faith. It is not unusual for the couple to be on different pages in one or more areas—their faith, their desire for children, timing for their family, etc. While this is not ideal, we encourage them to commit to unity as much as possible.

I'm going to break the prayer time into seven parts for you. While the prayer time is not rigid, but fluid, I've found that this structure works very well. Each part has a specific purpose and flows smoothly into the next part.

First: Interview the Woman or Couple

A typical prayer time starts with casual introductions and a short interview. We want everyone to feel comfortable and at ease. I assure everyone that this prayer time is totally confidential and no information will be shared outside the group. I always make sure to welcome the Holy Spirit to lead us during our hour. I just say a short prayer of "We welcome You, Holy Spirit." All team members have their Holy Spirit "antennae" up. This means we are all listening to God with our spiritual ears while tuning into the people with our physical ears. We interview the couple about their infertility history and any treatments they have tried. Keep this fairly short—probably no more than five minutes. Just the facts!

Second: Explain the Nature of Infertility and God's Desire to Cure It

Then I briefly explain the spiritual nature of infertility, stopping for questions and discussion if needed. I go on to make clear God's desire to cure infertility and bless couples with children. After I am sure the couple is aware of God's will, I explain how Satan often hinders conception. After about 20-30 minutes of sharing while we are listening both physically and spiritually, we are ready to pray. I assure the couple that we team members have faith for them. If they feel inadequate or weak in faith, I assure them we trust God's goodness and His will for them.

I inform all that we will ask the Holy Spirit to reveal any hindrance for them as a couple. I say something like, "Holy Spirit, show us any hindrance that is blocking this couple from receiving God's cure for their infertility and His gift of a child." Then we all listen.

Third: Listen to the Holy Spirit; Expose Hindrances

Listening to the Holy Spirit is where we depend on the gifts of the Holy Spirit. These gifts, noted earlier in this chapter, are for all believers and are God's supernatural help in ministry.

We remind the couple that God so wants to give them a child. We point out Satan lodged this hindrance in their path to thwart the will of God, that Satan is a defeated enemy, and that we have all power over him. We explain that once we expose Satan's stubborn obstacle, we can pray to remove it in Jesus's name. We assure each couple that what is a huge hindrance to one couple is of no significance to another. What may seem silly to one may be ultra-serious to another, so it is important to share what comes to mind.

If necessary, we may remind the couple that none of these hindrances can stop the truth that Jesus wiped out all their sin, even if they still struggle with sin. Sin is removed as far as the east is from the west by Jesus's work on the Cross. There is nothing they need to do to atone for their sin. Jesus did that. This is the Good News! He waits for them to agree.

We want the couple to hear from the Spirit concerning their specific hindrance, although the team members are also listening. I alert them to not think too hard and to be willing to share things that come to their minds that might not make sense to them or may seem embarrassing. In over 90 percent of the hundreds of prayer times I have led, the couple responds within about 45 seconds with a picture, a thought, or a memory. Often, they have the very same thought. We let them explain their sense of the hindrance. Team members may ask questions or add comments, sharing other pictures they saw or words that "popped" into their minds. These are all gifts of the Holy Spirit, such as a word of knowledge or wisdom or faith, that direct and empower our faith.

Fourth: Turn from Lies, Acknowledge God's Truth

Once a hindrance is identified, the team leads the couple in turning from believing lies to acknowledging God's truth. These lies or false beliefs might be concerning the power of Jesus's blood to remove all sin, or they might be lies about the desire of the Father to bless them with a child.

Perhaps they have harbored guilt from past sexual sin. Perhaps they have bitterness over a previous miscarriage or shame over a past abortion. Maybe they have believed a lie about God and His love or His desire to cure them. Sometimes, a woman who has a history of abortion or sexual disease does not think she is worthy to be a mother. She believes she does not meet God's qualifications. The truth is, Jesus qualifies her. Jesus makes her worthy. This is why Jesus died and rose again. He did what we cannot do—make ourselves worthy, holy, and righteous. With boldness, we proclaim Jesus has redeemed the woman from the curse that sin unleashed against her childbearing.

We help the couple turn (repent) from believing the lie that shame, guilt, or sin stops God. We help them know Jesus's work on the Cross was a mighty and complete success! We lead them to acknowledge this truth. All of this is done with simple prayers of "God, I am sorry for believing those lies. I now embrace your truth."

Fifth: Observe and Talk with the Couple

After praying about the hindrances, we observe and ask the couple if they experienced any physical sensations or if other thoughts have come to them. This might continue for 10 minutes or so. All the while, we listen to both the couple and to the Holy Spirit. Other team members might offer a thought or a picture. We usually pray again as the Spirit leads us.

Sixth: Pray for Healing

Once we are sure that any and all hindrances have been obliterated, we bless the couple with specific healing prayer. This is directed to any known physical or spiritual conditions that they have shared or the Spirit shows us. We like to follow the Biblical precedent of laying our hands on the people, if they agree to this. We believe the healing power of God flows through our hands, and so we ask for permission. This practice is spoken of in the Gospel of Mark:

> *They will be able to place their hands on the sick, and they will be healed (Mark 16:18).*

We lightly lay hands on them, being cautious to touch appropriately. Our faith is in Jesus, the Great Physician. We know He wants to flood their bodies with healing.

We bless the couple's sex life and ask God to unite the perfect egg and sperm. If a husband or wife has suffered a traumatic incident like sexual abuse or rape, we take time to invite the Spirit's healing of this deep, deep wound. These horrific violations against a person's body, mind, and emotions do real and painful damage. We pray as the Spirit leads so the person can be free of all damage, including freedom from shame, hatred, and rage. We pray the person is able to forgive those who have committed sins against him or her. Finally, we release God's cure for their infertility and ask for their child to be conceived.

Seventh: Bless the Couple

Once we determine that we have prayed for all the Spirit has highlighted, we conclude our team prayer with a prayer of blessing. Again, we listen to the Spirit to know how He specifically wants to speak encouragement and blessing to the couple. We usually affirm everything He has done, thank Him, and ask Him to seal and protect all that has happened during our prayer time.

An Example of Team Prayer

Charlotte was a lonely stay-at-home mom who starting attending church at the invitation of other moms she met at a local park. She was the mom of an active toddler, Tommy, and was thankful for a healthy son. But now, Charlotte confessed she battled discouraging secondary infertility. She had experienced four years of difficulty before conceiving Tommy, including a painful miscarriage. She was hopeful it would not be the same this time. However, after an active year of trying, she was not pregnant. Thoughts of another long struggle loomed over her.

Then she discovered we had prayer teams for infertility at our church. She was eager to receive prayer but had a gigantic concern. Ethan, her husband, was not a Christian and practiced another faith. He would not receive prayer. Would this sabotage her chance for prayer? Would we still pray for her? We assured her that although we like to have both husband and wife physically there together for prayer and on the same page spiritually, we were happy to pray even if Ethan would not come and even if he did not share the same faith. We gathered a team of three women and one man to pray and asked the Holy Spirit for His help.

God Shows Us How to Pray

While asking the Holy Spirit about hindrances, a team member saw a picture of Charlotte as a small girl. It was a time when she was filled with debilitating fear. When we asked her about this, Charlotte realized that she was still filled with fear, even as a grown woman. This unrelenting fear spilled over into so many aspects of her life and hindered her faith in God. We asked her to turn from this fear and choose to trust in Jesus. We spoke the truth that the Father's perfect love cleanses her of all fear. We allowed the Spirit to envelop her with the Father's unfailing love. She felt peaceful and free.

We then asked God to cure her infertility and give her another child. One team member received a word of prophetic encouragement for Charlotte. This is a type of prophecy where God reveals His great love, passion, care, provisions, and plans for others. God, speaking through a team member, assured her that she could relax, lavish love on her husband, and expect to be pregnant soon. One week later she was pregnant. A beautiful sister, Megan Marie, joined brother Tommy. Charlotte was overwhelmed with thankfulness when she discovered her secondary infertility was truly healed. Less than two years later, she conceived a third child with no problems at all. God loves to cure all infertility—including secondary infertility, too!

Team Prayer Review

Team prayer is so effective. So, gather a team of two to four others who are willing to set aside about an hour to meet and pray with the couple in a private setting without distractions. One person should lead the team by moving the prayer time along the seven steps. Here is a brief review of how to ask God together to cure infertility and give a child to an eager couple:

- Step One: Interview the couple.
- Step Two: Briefly explain infertility and God's desire to cure it.
- Step Three: Listen to the Spirit and expose hindrances.
- Step Four: Turn from lies and acknowledge God's truth.
- Step Five: Observe and talk with the couple about what they have experienced.
- Step Six: Pray for healing.
- Step Seven: Bless the couple.

We have used this basic model over and over again. Of course, it varies a bit with each couple, but the direction and content remain the same. It is so much fun to rejoice with the whole team when the couple finally announces: "We're pregnant!"

Julie's Journey

I want to conclude with sharing the rest of my daughter Julie's journey. I believe it illustrates that asking God for His cure is often a process and not a one-time event. After the year of no conception, a trip to the doctor confirmed her worst fears. She had PCOS, Polycystic Ovarian Syndrome. This explained her lack of menstrual periods and no ovulation.

Mike and Julie faced their crisis of infertility by immediately asking God for His cure and His gift of a child. They sensed God was instructing them to rely on Him as He directed their choices. Medically, they opted for Julie to take Metformin to correct her insulin levels and treat the PCOS. This was the easy part. Of course, Julie expected quick results. She began taking the drug and started calculating the best month to give birth.

Watch Out for "Perfect Timing"

They, like many other couples, had figured the perfect timing for conception and birth. Julie was a teacher in the public schools and just knew the end of May would be great for giving birth. She would have the whole Midwest summer to enjoy with her newborn. When August, September, October, and November passed without the pregnancy test reading positive, she was devastated. She thought she had "heard from God." This is a common mistake for couples whose personal pain clouds their ability to hear the voice of God. Our own deep desires drown Him out. This is why we need others praying, counseling, and helping us keep our hearts and minds clear to hear God. They received powerful team prayer several times and exposed some hindrances where Satan was lying about God's timing. He had convinced Julie it would be long, like Sarah in the Bible, who waited 25 years. She saw this was not true and turned from this lie and her despair.

Jealousy Hinders

Another major hindrance for Julie was her battle with jealousy. Any time a friend or relative announced a pregnancy, Julie found herself thinking: "Oh, no, where is mine?" Anger, jealousy, and hopelessness would be stirred up again, followed by a sense that somehow the supply of babies was diminishing and she was missing out.

As ludicrous as that sounds now, it was a powerful lie the enemy lodged in Julie's mind. When she saw friend after friend and even strangers conceive, she calculated her chances as rapidly disappearing. It was especially difficult that fall, as two close sisters-in-law were both pregnant. She faced more baby showers where she would have to spend the time forcing a smile while inwardly she raged. She knew we had to ask God about this destructive force in her heart.

Rejoice with Others

She realized she believed the lie that God's will for curing infertility and blessing with children did not really apply to her. As Julie and I talked and prayed about this, she acknowledged that she believed these lies about God and about His love for her as His daughter. She admitted she knew in her heart He wanted to bless her and that He loved her deeply and had a baby for her. She made a decision to instantly rejoice when she received the news of another's pregnancy. This was not easy. But rejoicing with others and thanking God for the upcoming blessing released fresh faith into Julie's heart.

God Reveals Timing

We continued to ask God to speak, while thanking Him for His cure and the gift of a child. One day while I was reading again the story of Sarah in the Bible, God showed me a phrase the angel spoke about Sarah and I knew it was for Julie. I told her I believed God was saying "at this time next year" (November 2008) she would be holding a baby—the same words the angel had spoken about Sarah. I emphasized that nothing is too hard for the Lord and He was speaking to her, giving her the chance to trust Him and His timing. She knew in her heart that this was God speaking, too. She and Mike rested in faith.

> Sure enough, by mid-December, Julie called me one morning at 5:20 a.m. In a deep sleep, I heard the startling ring of the phone pierce the silence. I jumped to answer with my heart pounding. "Mom," she said excitedly, "I think the test says I'm pregnant!" Immediately I was awake, joy flooding my soul! Indeed she was.

"I'm Pregnant!"

Sure enough, by mid-December, Julie called me one morning at 5:20 a.m. In a deep sleep, I heard the startling ring of the phone pierce the silence. I jumped to answer with my heart pounding. "Mom," she said excitedly, "I think the test says I'm pregnant!" Immediately I was awake, joy flooding my soul! Indeed she was. Three more pregnancy tests—later that day—confirmed the miraculous truth. After 15 months of trying, she was pregnant. Ty Michael Yoder was born August 28, 2008, and Julie was definitely holding him in her arms in November 2008—a year from the time God had shown us she would be cradling a newborn. Julie has since had two more beautiful children. Tate Christopher took a little time to conceive in 2010, but Julie is completely healed of PCOS. Magdalena Marie, conceived in 2013, was a surprise and a reminder of God's amazing, miraculous love.

Ask!

So, ask God. Ask with confidence and boldness. Because, now you know how to pray. Now you can invite others to pray with you, too. Now you can be sure God hears you and delights to give you the deepest desire of your hearts. God wants to talk with you on how to receive His cure. Ask Him! And if your faith begins to waver, the next chapter has wisdom on strengthening your belief and being assured of God's love and blessing for you.

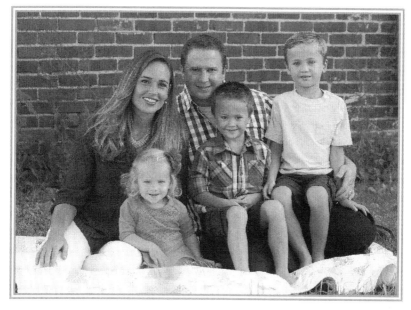

Julie, Mike, Maggie, Tate, and Ty Yoder

Important Truths for Your Journey

- Prayer is simply talking to God—in this case, about the deepest desire of your heart.
- God hears and answers prayer.
- God wants you to pray in faith.
- Joining with others is a powerful way to pray.
- The Holy Spirit will direct your prayer time.

Recommended Actions Steps

- Ask God! He wants to give you His cure and your child. Ask God to reveal any hindrances. Review Chapter 5 on hindrances and ask God to show you any hindrances in your situation. Usually, these are incidences in our lives that have caused us to believe lies about God's love, goodness, and forgiveness. The action step is to repent—or turn from—these lies and embrace the truth. Listen for those things that pop in your mind. Do not dredge up your past! When you think you know a hindrance, ask God to remove it and show you truth.
- Pray! Ask out loud together with your spouse for God's cure and your child. Ask, knowing God is a good Father who wants to give you good things, including His cure for infertility and the gift of a child.
- Write out your prayer so you can revisit it daily to affirm your faith in God's love for you and His ability to cure you and to thank God for His answer.
- Listen for God's specific instructions to you in areas of concern. Talk with Him about any questions or concerns. Ask for His wisdom. When thoughts pop in your head or Bible verses come to mind, know this is possibly God speaking to you. Rarely do you hear an audible voice, but you might! Also, be alert for the Lord to speak to you through dreams.
- Do be careful of any negative input. Satan is the father of lies and will attempt to fill your mind with negative information and thoughts. Stay away from the Internet if reading blogs or info sites discourages you. Guard your heart and mind.
- Definitely consider gathering a small team to pray with you. This is so powerful and so encouraging. Follow the simple steps for praying together.

Chapter 7

Believing God for the Impossible

"We are confused about believing when we cannot see."

Lindy and Ben are both very attractive thirty-something professionals with young, already successful careers. Lindy owns a popular fitness and nutrition business, while Ben works in banking and finance. They are the epitome of hard work, dedication, and motivation. They are a power couple on the move. Ben and Lindy are used to getting things done and are experts at expending much effort, and they applied this same mode to generating faith for pregnancy. However, after several years of trying to get pregnant, their hard work, dedication, and motivation did not result in the same success as it did in their careers. Frustrated and anxious, they met with a team to pray and listen for God's instructions.

Listening

As always, we knew God's will was to bless them with a child. We now waited to hear what needed to be prayed in their specific situation. While we listened to their story, our team saw that Lindy and Ben had tried with all their might to produce faith for a child. We saw how they had subtly taken their eyes off Jesus and His desire to give them a child and had focused on themselves and their own efforts. They were exhausted with no results. Their hard work had thwarted faith in Jesus and replaced it with faith in themselves. As we listened to them and to God, we sensed they were trying to do something only God can do. He alone produces faith.

Faith is Important

Maybe you, like Lindy and Ben, have tried to produce faith that pleases God. You might be exhausted with no results, and now you are somewhat confused about faith. How do you have faith for the impossible? Where does it come from? What is this "rest of faith"? These are good questions, and God's Word has much to say about faith.

Faith is obviously very important to God. Faith is at the core of our relationship with Him:

> *And without faith it is impossible to please him, for whoever would draw near to God must believe that he exists and that he rewards those who seek him (Hebrews 11:6).*

Faith pleases God. We are in relationship with God by faith. We live by faith. We walk by faith. Faith is essential to a healthy, fruitful relationship with Jesus. It is the prayer of faith that has power to move mountains. It is the prayer of faith that God hears and answers. No question about it, when it comes to our relationship with the Living God, faith is crucial! The Father loves faith.

God is Faithful

When we know God is faithful, it anchors our faith. And God is faithful! God's faithfulness to us and to His promises abounds throughout both the Old and New Testaments; His faithfulness is a common thread that binds all of Scripture together.

And our faith in God is critical. It changes our worldview and opens up possibilities we would have never before seen or believed in. Faith was so vital in 90-year-old, infertile Sarah's conception of Isaac:

> *By faith Sarah herself received power to conceive, even when she was past the age, since she considered him faithful who had promised. Therefore from one man, and him as good as dead, were born descendants as many as the*

stars of heaven and as many as the innumerable grains of sand by the sea-shore (Hebrews 11:11-12).

She considered God faithful. That is the essence of real faith. God *is* faithful! This is what you need to know and what you need to believe. However, there are distorted teachings on faith and misunderstandings that harm faith.

Misconceptions About Faith

One of the most destructive teachings about faith that I have experienced (and witnessed in Lindy and Ben) is that somehow we have to produce faith, enough faith, to move God's hand to answer our prayers. While the teaching may not be stated as such, the sense one gets is that we are responsible for this commodity of faith. We try really hard to believe. We quote Scriptures. We meditate on the Word. We try to move the hand of God, so we listen intently to God's Word. We study the Bible and speak it out because we know faith comes by hearing God's Word:

So faith comes from hearing, and hearing through the word of Christ (Romans 10:17).

Once we have somehow garnered a specific (and unknown) amount of faith through listening, reading, and speaking the Word, this faith is offered to God as "payment," and we wait for our request to be answered—as if God were a clerk in a store and we could walk up to the counter and plunk down our faith to purchase our fertility! That's not how He works, and that's not how faith works.

If we have embraced this teaching on faith, then when prayers are not answered, we are left feeling like a failure. We failed to have enough faith to please God. We feel guilty and in despair. We don't know what to do. Without acknowledging it, we have tried to manufacture faith.

Failed Faith

If we have embraced this teaching on faith, then when prayers are not answered, we are left feeling like a failure. We failed to have enough faith to please God. We feel guilty and in despair. We don't know what to do. Without acknowledging it, we have tried to manufacture faith. We may have said Bible verses out loud, trying to create faith in our heart for the much-wanted pregnancy. Or maybe we buy another maternity top to show God that we have faith since faith without action or "works" is dead:

So also faith by itself, if it does not have works, is dead. (James 2:17).

What are the "works" that indicate living faith? We are told to show our faith by our works, to show God we believe Him. We may find ourselves saying, "Do you see my faith, God? Is this enough faith, God? Do I believe strongly enough now, God?" We say these words in our hearts as we work hard to believe. But this faith fails. It fails because it is essentially "faith in our own faith"!

Please do not misunderstand me. It is very important to meditate on the Word. It is very important to confess the Scriptures. It is very important to have faith with accompanying action. But none of these produce faith per se. Not the God kind of faith. Not the faith that pleases God. Not faith for the impossible.

Faith is in Jesus, Not in Ourselves

The faith we want and need is *not* in our own faith or our own ability to produce faith. No. A thousand times no. That is actually pagan religion. Pagans offer all kinds of sacrifices, incantations, and even their own children to appease their gods and get what they hope to get—rain, fertility, protection, etc. When we try to muster up faith and offer our puny attempts to believe and not doubt, we are relying on self-effort and on our own works. This is in direct contradiction to the Gospel, which reveals the amazing work of Jesus on the Cross and His invitation to trust Him. The first lesson we must learn when it comes to faith is that our faith is in a Person, Jesus. Our faith is in Him and His love for us and His work of healing on our behalf. Our faith is in His invitation to ask Him and trust Him. Our faith is not in ourselves. Our faith for the impossible is in Jesus.

Jesus is the author and finisher of our faith. This means that He is the One who ignites faith in our hearts. He produces faith in us and we simply acknowledge it and receive it.

Jesus is the Author of Our Faith

Jesus is the author and finisher of our faith. This means that He is the One who ignites faith in our hearts. He produces faith in us and we simply acknowledge it and receive it. He is eager for us to do so. Our faith is in Him, and He lives inside us. We keep our "eyes" on Him. We look to Him:

> Looking unto Jesus the author and finisher of our faith . . . (Hebrews 12:2).

Jesus releases faith in our hearts. He wants to help our unbelief and give us faith for the impossible. He wants us first and foremost to have faith in His love and His willingness to cure us and give us a child. Jesus delights in being the author of faith in our hearts. Jesus often referenced people's faith in Him and how powerful this faith was. When we read these stories, He brings faith to our hearts.

Jesus Heals by Faith

Faith is especially prominent in many of Jesus's healings. Sometimes, Jesus commends the person for having faith, as He did the woman who had bled for twelve years:

> And behold, a woman who had suffered from a discharge of blood for twelve years came up behind him and touched the fringe of his garment, for she said to herself, "If I only touch his garment, I will be made well." Jesus turned, and seeing her he said, "Take heart, daughter; your faith has made you well." And instantly the woman was made well (Matthew 9:20-22).

She was a despised outcast among her people, the Jews, and should not have been in public with a blood discharge. She took a dangerous risk to venture out. Her actual life was at stake when she dared to touch Jesus, a holy Rabbi, and infect Him with her uncleanness. But, oh, what faith she had. Was it faith in her ability to be great, perfect, and strong? No! A hundred times no! Her faith was in Jesus—the One she had heard did miracles for the last, the least, and the lost. She timidly touched His robe, and miraculous healing coursed through her weak and ailing body. This was her way of asking Jesus for His cure for her sickness. Her faith had made her whole—her faith in Jesus. You, too, can have this simple, but powerful, faith in the God who loves you. Ask Him right now to release faith in your heart.

Believe God is Love

Our faith is in our faithful, loving God. This was a very important breakthrough for me as I waited for Jesus to bless us with the conception of our first child. I was worshipping Him one day, just singing to Him, and trying to talk with Him about my impatience. I was asking Him how was I going to persevere and have a faith that really pleased Him, without doubt of any kind. He told me to read Hebrews 11:6 again. I was so familiar with this passage that I was almost insulted. But I grabbed my Bible and read the passage I had read hundreds of times in the past few months.

> *And without faith it is impossible to please Him, for he who comes to God must believe that He is . . . (Hebrews 11:6 NASB).*

And this is where He stopped me and said, "How do you finish that sentence, Dianne?" Believe He is . . . I had always taken this to mean I was to believe that God exists, that He is real, as that's what comes through in other translations. And while that is true—God *is* real—suddenly I saw that passage differently. When prodded by Jesus to "finish that sentence," I saw that God is first and foremost LOVE. Yes, that is what His Word says:

> *Beloved, let us love one another, for love is from God, and whoever loves has been born of God and knows God. Anyone who does not love does not know God, because God is love (1 John 4:7-8).*

God is *love*. He said He wanted me to believe that He is love. He wanted me to believe that His love for me knows no bounds. He wanted me to know that I could trust His love for me. He of course wanted to give me a child because He loved me—not because I had such great faith or strong faith or enough faith. Did I believe that? Yes. And right then, as I trusted His unfailing love for me, I know Jesus released fresh faith in my heart.

Receive God's Love in Worship

One of the best ways to have this fresh faith released in your heart and to connect more and more with the Father's love for you is through worship. Pouring out your heart to God through song cultivates an intimacy with God that is rich and deep. God wants you to know His perfect love that drives all fear out of your heart.

> *There is no fear in love, but perfect love casts out fear . . . We love because He first loved us (1 John 4:18, 19).*

My whole life radically changed when I discovered worship. Suddenly, singing *to* God, not just *about* Him, empowered me to draw close to Him and express my love for Him in new and transforming ways. Finally, I knew how to do what Psalm 37 invites us to do:

> *Delight yourself in the* LORD, *and he will give you the desires of your heart* (Psalm 37:4).

Yes! Now I more readily believed God would grant me the dearest desire of my heart—the desire for a baby. I received His love for me. I gave my love back to Him.

Worship Strengthens Faith

Worship not only *released* faith in me; it also *strengthened* faith. Worship forever changed me! I have found personal, intimate worship to be one of the best ways to strengthen faith and soak in the Father's unchanging and unfailing love for me. You can make the choice to let the Father love you. Worship is helpful in dismantling our fears, confusion, impatience, and weariness. Through worship, you can choose to trust His love and receive His love. You can be healed by His love. This is a very important part of your journey of faith.

Faith actually works by love. Worship will make a huge difference as you wait for your child. Worship gets your eyes off your own circumstances and onto Jesus. See Appendix D for suggested worship resources, begin to build your playlist, and experience the transforming power of Jesus's love for you. Faith for the impossible will rise in your heart.

Another lesson in faith I learned was how to receive in faith. When Happy and I prayed, God wanted us to know and believe that we had already received our answer to the prayer. He wanted us to trust we had it now. He wanted us to stop repeatedly asking and begin to thank Him every day for our baby.

Believe and Receive

Another lesson in faith I learned was how to receive in faith. When Happy and I prayed, God wanted us to know and believe that we had already received our answer to the prayer. He wanted us to trust we had it now. He wanted us to stop repeatedly asking and begin to thank Him every day for our baby. I had some questions about this! Trust that I was pregnant now? But, I wasn't! At least my body did not know it. Hmm . . . What was this lesson in faith? Mark wrote one of the Scriptures the Spirit used to teach us about praying in faith:

> *Therefore I say to you, whatever things you ask when you pray, believe that you receive them, and you will have them (Mark 11:24).*

We had asked for our healing and for a child to be conceived. The Spirit wanted us to believe that we had received our healthy conception and to be assured that in due time, we would see proof. This did coincide with the definition of faith found in Hebrews 11:

> *Now faith is the substance of things hoped for, the evidence of things not seen (Hebrews 11:1).*

According to this definition, faith means believing in what you can't yet see. True, we could not see any pregnancy or any sign of pregnancy. But by faith we had received our healing and knew it would eventually result in a baby. Did this seem a bit awkward or did it feel like we were faking it? Yes, sometimes it did. But the Spirit taught us so many valuable lessons from the Word about how faith in God works.

Abraham's Lesson: Don't Look at Your Body!

Abraham taught me one important lesson about receiving by faith. Here is a description of how Abraham responded to God's promise:

> *As it is written, "I have made you (Abraham) a father of many nations" . . . in the presence of Him whom he believed—God, who gives life to the dead and calls those things which do not exist as though they did; who, contrary to hope, in hope believed . . . And not being weak in faith, he did not consider his own body, already dead (since he was about a hundred years old), and the deadness of Sarah's womb. He did not waver at the promise of God through unbelief, but was strengthened in faith, giving glory to God, and being fully convinced that what He had promised He was also able to perform (Romans 4:16-21).*

I saw how Abraham did not consider his own dead body or the deadness of Sarah's womb. He did not pay attention to the natural circumstances and physical evidence. They all screamed, *Impossible!* Instead, by faith he looked at the promise of God. He was convinced God was able to do what He had said. God had said Abraham would be the father of many. He said Abraham and Sarah would have their own son. This was what they focused on. Abraham was fully convinced and gave glory to God. He and Sarah did not waver through unbelief.

Yes! That was how I would live. I would not look at my own body, now considered medically dead as far as ever reproducing. I would not be checking for physical signs every minute of the day. I would not tune into: "Do my breasts feel tender? Am I going to the bathroom more? Do I feel a bit nauseous? Should I take a pregnancy test?" No! These were all things I had done repeatedly for the three years I was specifically dealing with our infertility. Looking at my body had done nothing but discourage and depress me. No. I decided not to consider my own body, now dead.

Listen for God's Instructions to You

Look to God. Listen for Him. Look to the promises of God and don't waver in unbelief. Choose to believe His Word. These are all actions I had to intentionally take. I knew he had heard my prayer and had answered. I would choose to thank Him every day. I would choose to give glory to God for blessing us with a baby. I would have faith for the impossible—faith in God.

This is just one illustration of how God will talk with you after you have asked Him for His cure. He wants to help you to believe you have received your answer from Him, even if you do not yet see it. This is faith in God. You trust His timing but meanwhile, you listen for thoughts that pop in your head, Bible references to read or reread, even others' words of wisdom that strengthen you. Then, you choose how to "receive and rest in faith" together as husband and wife. Every couple is different in how God will work with them and strengthen their faith for the impossible while they wait. God will show you how to believe you have received His cure. All of this will enable you to persevere in faith.

Perseverance is Vital to Faith

Perseverance is another vital aspect of faith for the impossible. Of course, we live in the 21st century, and we do not like to wait for anything—even a five-minute wait at the drive-through makes us antsy. But God is ready to empower us to persevere. Jesus knows and shows us where we need strength, and helps us to persevere when we start to doubt or get discouraged. When we struggle with impatience or are tempted to give up, we can ask the Father to strengthen us by His Spirit. This is a good prayer to pray:

> *For this reason I bow my knees before the Father, from whom every family in heaven and on earth is named, that according to the riches of his glory he may grant you to be strengthened with power through his Spirit in your inner being (Ephesians 3:14-16).*

He loves to answer this prayer. In the fullness of His time, He will release exactly what you need. Hold on to that. You will have faith for the impossible.

Meditate on Scriptures

Meanwhile, it is helpful to meditate on the Scriptures that speak the most to you. Have these on your phone or posted on your mirror. These are not just words. These are God's words—to you! Read and believe them. I have listed some of my favorite Scriptures in Appendix C, but please find the ones that are most meaningful to you. These remind you that God is faithful and He has a baby for you. Remember, too, that this is a relationship with the One who knows us better than we know ourselves. He speaks to us in His Word, highlighting meaningful, personal Scriptures for us to reflect on. He faithfully unveils our misconceptions. He lovingly corrects us and moves us ahead. Our journey is often plagued by doubt, but God reveals what we need to know to be free of doubt and grow in faith for the impossible.

Don't Be Deceived About Doubt

Doubt can debilitate us. Doubt plays tricks on our minds. Doubt can be so deceptive. We can think doubt ruins faith for the impossible. We try hard not to doubt. Jesus tells us we should not doubt:

> *So Jesus answered and said to them, "Have faith in God. For assuredly, I say to you, whoever says to this mountain, 'Be removed and be cast into the sea,' and does not doubt in his heart, but believes that those things he says will be done, he will have whatever he says. Therefore I say to you, whatever things you ask when you pray, believe that you receive them, and you will have them" (Mark 11:22-24).*

This is powerful faith that moves mountains, even the mountain of infertility. But, no doubt in our heart? How do we do that?

Lessons on Doubt

I learned some valuable lessons about doubt as I was battling it daily while I waited to experience God's cure. I had read this Mark 11 passage about believing and not doubting. I had read the Romans 4:20 passage that said Abraham did not doubt. I was determined not to doubt. But I battled doubt continually. Satan daily lied to me, giving me plenty of opportunities to doubt. As I was talking to Jesus about my doubt one day, He told me to read the entire story of Abraham and Sarah found in Genesis.

As I was reading this account I saw, for the first time, how Abraham obviously doubted God's promise to him. Abraham knew he was to have an heir as God had said, but when it did not happen with his wife Sarah, he took Sarah's maid, Hagar, and conceived a child, Ishmael. It was doubt that compelled Abraham to go to Hagar when Sarah was not getting pregnant. But, this son, Ishmael, was not God's promise to him and was evidence of Abraham's doubt. Of course, God did not disqualify Abraham because of this doubt. No. God kept talking with him and leading him to trust God's promise. I saw I had good company in the world of doubt. Doubt was normal, and God can handle it and show us how to deal with it.

Doubt Busters

I needed to bust the doubt in my heart. Or, more accurately, I needed God to bust the doubt in my heart! We are in partnership with God and we cooperate with His life in us. So, I carefully wrote out all the promises on 3x5 notecards to repeat them out loud every day. This was in addition to the prayer I had written earlier. These written reminders helped dissipate doubt when it wanted to creep back up in my heart.

Another powerful doubt buster for me was speaking God's Word out loud. Words have power. Words can change things. This is a truth revealed over and over in Scripture. God created through His spoken word. Confession of the truth brought faith to my heart and released faith for the impossible. With boldness, we proclaimed God's gift of a baby to us. Sometimes we spoke this to others. Sometimes we just spoke this ourselves, to our bodies and to our hearts. The spoken word of God has power. Faith for the impossible came to our hearts.

Deal with Your Doubt

God will faithfully expose your doubt and instruct you what to do. Be honest with Him about your doubt. Do not deny it. Do not hide it. Do not be deceived by its offers of substitutes tempting to you rename your doubt as "being humble" or "open to what God wants" instead of just admitting doubt and asking for help.

> *Be alert for how God directs you to deal with doubt. He may nudge you to read certain Bible accounts. He may impress you to stop listening to certain friends or some Internet voices. He might show you certain Scripture verses to read and speak out. Speaking God's Word is one of many different instructions the Spirit may give to you.*

Be alert for how God directs you to deal with doubt. He may nudge you to read certain Bible accounts. He may impress you to stop listening to certain friends or some Internet voices. He might show you certain Scripture verses to read and speak out. Speaking God's Word is one of many different instructions the Spirit may give to you. While it may feel funny at first, you may discover just how powerful confession of God's Word really is. It is dynamite that destroys the lies of the enemy and releases faith in God's goodness and healing. God wants you to have faith for the impossible, and He will help you overcome doubt. Choose to obey what you sense Him telling you!

Choices Can Be Difficult

Choices can be difficult, especially when our physical senses scream the opposite of what we are choosing to believe and do. It can feel like we are fake or trying to prove something to God. Make sure your faith is in Him, not in your own choices or actions. Our faith is in a Person, God Himself. We are in a loving relationship with Him. He knows our hearts. He hears our cries. He answers our prayers.

The Spirit is faithful to show you what actions to take. He will enable you to step out in faith, not in fear or in faking it. He wants you to experience the joy of answered prayer. He wants you to be sure of God's faithfulness. He does not want you worried about your own faith. He is faithful to do as He says. He will give you faith like a grain of mustard seed, faith for the impossible. As Jesus says:

> *"For truly, I say to you, if you have faith like a grain of mustard seed, you will say to this mountain, 'Move from here to there,' and it will move, and nothing will be impossible for you" (Matthew 21:20).*

Faith moves mountains. Faith destroys the impossible. You only need a mustard seed of faith. Jesus is so ready to give this to you. He is not pleased when you try to produce this yourselves. Again, your faith is in Him. He is ready to move the mountain of infertility out of your life. He is ready for that seed of faith to produce the fruit of a child.

God will show each of you how to walk in faith. He will show you where doubt has deceived you. He will fill your hearts with His faith—a faith that triumphs over doubt. The "rest" of faith is so important to our Father; He wants to give this to you so you are at peace and are not afraid. Jesus will make sure you reach your destination of motherhood—in His timing.

Trust God for His Timing

Timing is one of the most difficult aspects of waiting in faith. It is hard to trust God for His timing. It is especially hard when we are waiting month by month to see if the "magic has happened." Of course, we so often think our timing is the right timing. We figure things out in our heads and note that, "Yes, September would be the perfect month to have a baby." It fits in with our work schedules, our commitments, the seasonal weather, and so many other facets we are sure make a huge difference in giving birth. We let God know all of this, trying to convince Him to move.

Over and over I have watched hopes be dashed as the critical month of conception has come and gone. Despair sets in once again as the "perfect month" has passed—again.

God knows the perfect timing for your baby's birth. He is often waiting for us—waiting for us to trust Him for His timing and to stop our bargaining and our weak attempts to manipulate Him. When we are willing to surrender our timing, our schedules, our control, to Him, we not only rest in faith, but we also activate His timing. We can hear His voice and follow His lead. We are not in charge. He is.

Receiving the Proclamation

Mother's Day, which of course always falls on a Sunday, is a tough day for infertile couples, especially the women. It is another cruel, albeit unintentional, reminder that their arms are empty, their prayers unanswered. They are not yet mothers. I know many women refuse to worship on Mother's Day because the focus is often on celebrating mothers and honoring their love and sacrifice. I am super sensitive to this as a pastor. I, too, often dreaded Mother's Day.

On Mother's Day 2014, after I finished preaching, I instructed women who were waiting for God to bless their wombs to stand. I wanted to take this time to pray over them. I wanted to acknowledge their pain and give them fresh hope in God. It took courage for some just to stand. The humiliation of infertility compels one to hide. About five women stood, some with their husbands. Lindy and her husband, Ben, were one of the couples standing to receive prayer. Of course, we had already prayed for them several times and there had been no progress to date.

After a brief prayer, I sensed the Holy Spirit telling me to take a big risk. I said, "I feel strongly that God is instructing me to say this today and that it is meant for someone specific. It's always a little scary when this happens, to step out and make a bold statement like this, but I feel it's what I'm supposed to do. God knows your hurt and your longing and he has great blessings in store for you." I continued, "He wants you to know that *at this time next year, you will be holding a son!*"

Lindy later shared this on Facebook: "When I heard Di's words, my eyes immediately filled with tears (they still do now as I tell it), and I got chills. I truly believed in that moment that she was talking directly to me, and that her words were meant for me. I just knew it. I received the proclamation that next year at this time, on Mother's Day, I would be holding a son."

The Holy Spirit Releases Faith for the Impossible

This is often how the Holy Spirit works. We respond in faith, and the next thing we know, we don't have to "manufacture" belief; we really believe. We just know a prayer or a word that was spoken is for us. We receive it. However, now the waiting begins.

Lindy continued with her story: "Then, May and June both passed with negative pregnancy test results. I began to doubt and get upset with God. I believed those words! I wanted them to be for me. Why isn't it happening? If it is going to be next year in May, it needs to happen now! And then, in July—a positive test. It was the last month I could've gotten those results in time for a baby to arrive before Mother's Day."

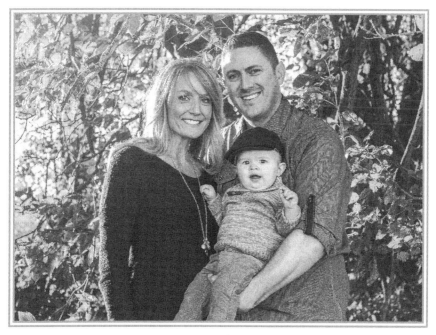

Lindy, Ben, and Lincoln Gault

A Son?

Of course, Lindy and Ben were thrilled. But . . . would it be a son they were holding? Thanks to modern sonograms, they were able to post on Facebook that this miracle baby was indeed a boy. And Lincoln Thomas arrived safe and sound on Saturday, April 4, 2015, his exact due date, and just in time for Mother's Day 2015. His overjoyed mama reported, "My labor was complication-free, and we went home just 24 hours later. Lincoln is simply amazing. He's a happy, smiling baby, and we regularly get comments on his peaceful nature. We are so blessed!"

Believe Words of Encouragement

All of us are so thankful for God's goodness, faithfulness, and timing. It is so helpful to receive words of encouragement. Did you note how Lindy believed those words were for her and she grabbed them into her heart? Again, the Holy Spirit strengthened her faith. She received those words. Faith in God, not her own faith, moved her mountain of infertility.

I really cannot explain how this happens. Nor would I ever tell anyone to try and "make it happen." But, I can tell you God wants your faith to be strengthened. He wants to speak to you. He wants to give you mountain-moving faith. So be alert. Be listening. Most of all, He wants to give you the desire of your heart—in the fullness of His time.

What If Nothing Happens?

However, I would be remiss if I did not address the very pressing question of: "What if I received such encouragement and felt it was God and then I was let down again, devastated when I did not conceive, and the words spoken to me were obviously false. What if nothing happens?" That is so hard. That really tests our faith and our ability to keep on trusting God. We feel foolish. We feel tricked. We feel devastated once again. The pain is very real. It seems unusually cruel. We ask, "Why God?"

While I do not know how each of you feels in these situations, I know how horrible this was for me on several occasions. Copious tears were shed time and time again. Screams were unleashed at God. Doubt threatened to abort even the tiniest seed of faith.

Yet, in my darkness, the Light of Jesus was still there. And as I asked Him to show me what was going on, He was faithful to do so.

Yet, in my darkness, the Light of Jesus was still there. And as I asked Him to show me what was going on, He was faithful to do so. One time I saw that I had just flat out not heard God like I thought and while it was confusing and hurtful, I was still loved and cared for by God. Another time, a person shared a well-meaning, but nevertheless inaccurate, impression with me about the timing of my hoped-for pregnancy. When it became apparent that it was not true, I had to forgive her and realign my trust in God.

Most importantly during these tough times, Jesus always reassured me that He had not forgotten my prayer for a child and I could know my answer would come. I could count on Him to repair my damaged faith, bring fresh strength to my weary body, and work in my heart faith for the impossible. He is a faithful God!

Important Truths for Your Journey

- Our faith is in Jesus, not in ourselves or in our ability to believe. We trust Him.
- We can strengthen our faith through worship, where we grow in our love for God and His love for us.
- God will show us how to receive by faith and put our faith into action.
- We can face doubt and deal with it as God tells us.
- God will release faith for the impossible into our hearts.
- We can surrender our timetables and control to God, trusting His way.
- God will help us through every difficult circumstance.

Recommended Action Steps

- Talk to God about your doubts and fears.
- Download a worship playlist and play it regularly.
- Make a list of Scriptures to meditate on.

Chapter 8

Partnering with Your Spouse and with God

"Are there things we can do to cooperate with God or do we just wait?"

Sometimes God surprises us with answers that seem "out of the blue." I have witnessed and heard of more than a few astounding and quick answers to prayer for infertility, where a couple who has been waiting a long while to conceive and has encountered many obstacles, suddenly gets healed in response to a one-time prayer for them.

Jenna and Jack had tried for four years to have a child. While there were a few minor physical issues, both were healthy, and they should have had no trouble conceiving. But, month after month passed with no baby in sight. One night they were attending a special meeting where the teacher shared on healing. At the close of the service, the speaker said God had shown him there were five infertile couples in the audience. He asked them to come forward for prayer. He said God would heal them. Jenna and Jack jumped to their feet and ran forward to receive prayer. It was a simple, three-second prayer. There were no unusual feelings, no spectacular displays. Ten months later Benjamin Mark was born.

I love when God surprises couples this way. I pray some of you reading this are blessed with such a delightful surprise. However, these answers to prayer are somewhat unpredictable. Often, couples are waiting and wondering what to do.

A Way Forward

I want to make sure you have a way forward in your present pain. You have learned how to pray to God and how to believe God in your journey to receive God's cure for infertility. You still face some obstacles ahead. But, all obstacles are opportunities to grow in your relationship with God. No obstacle is too great for Him. You are ready to take that third step of reinforcing your partnership with your spouse and with God. God is more than ready to remove all obstacles as you listen, obey, and delight in your partnership with Him and with one another. Following are some issues to consider and steps you can carry out as you partner with God and each other while you wait.

Sometimes men can feel isolated and unsure of their role in the process. The desire for a baby can become an idol in a woman's life and she can fail to see the value of her husband and to show him love and appreciation. Yet, this is a team effort, and healthy partnership is essential.

Husband-Wife Dynamics

The cooperation between husband and wife is one of the most important dynamics when it comes to receiving God's cure for infertility. Sometimes men can feel isolated and unsure of their role in the process. The desire for a baby can become an idol in a woman's life, and she can fail to see the value of her husband, and thus struggle to show him love and appreciation. Yet, this is a team effort, and healthy partnership is essential.

More Than a Sperm Donor?

"I'm trying hard to be supportive of my wife through this struggle," Andrew lamented. "But, at times it feels like I am nothing more than a sperm donor. We barely have sex anymore because we are in the middle of another procedure and we need to concentrate on that. Frankly, it's not always easy providing samples for these. Before that, when we did have sex, it was so monitored for the exact right time and she wanted it to be so quick, I didn't even enjoy it. I can't believe I am saying this. But it's true. My emotions are pretty wasted. My manhood is reduced to shreds. Is all of this really worth it? I am really beginning to doubt."

He shook his head and sighed deeply. I sat in silence for a moment, letting the gravity of his words sink in. I knew how difficult it was for this young, strong, healthy-looking husband to bare his soul in my presence. I knew how much he loved his wife, Kate, and how much he yearned to make everything okay. I also knew his suffering was real, yet often ignored. It reminded me again how important it is to pay attention to the husband and his needs and concerns on this journey towards God's cure for infertility. Men do matter, and the partnership of husband and wife is critical. Men are more than a sperm donor.

Men Are Important in This Struggle

I am well aware that the primary audience for this book is women. However, men are a vital part of this struggle. I mean, without the guys, there surely would be no baby! Many men feel helpless when it comes to comforting their wife month after disappointing month. Her emotions of despair and frustration leave her husband feeling like a failure. Oh, yes, the husband is doing his part . . . but even sex is a drag when it is demanded at the worst and most inconvenient times.

Some of you might identify with Andrew's sentiments. Some men have even struggled to "perform" due to the pressure of "we have to do it right now." Then there are the endless rounds of doctor appointments, drugs, and procedures. Not to mention the absolute drain on the bank account for those who do not have adequate insurance. How can men and women partner in this journey of receiving God's cure for infertility?

First, men, realize that yes, you are much more than just a sperm donor! As important as that is, there are several critical contributions you make in this journey of healing and hope. You are a loving husband and soon-to-be father. Your partnership in marriage, in prayer, and in faith is foundational. Your own physical, emotional, and spiritual health is a key factor in maintaining a balanced and healthy relationship with your wife. Your opinion in areas of timing, finances, and medical procedures is likewise important. It is essential that you and your wife can discuss things freely and are in general agreement about the decisions you are making for your family. In addition, your awareness of and confession of possible spiritual hindrances can make a big difference in the conception of a child. Cooperation between you and your wife makes a huge difference. These are such significant roles as you journey hand in hand with your wife.

Men Are Prominent in Bible Accounts

God's first command to be fruitful and multiply was given to both husband and wife. (So, guys, definitely have lots of sex!) The Bible also shows the prominence that men have in the journey of infertility. Infertility plays such a dominant role in the unfolding of God's Story of Redemption, starting with Abraham, the infertile father of our faith. He was given the promise of an heir whose birth would unleash the multiplication of a new people, a people of God.   He was an old man—100 years old to be exact—and his wife Sarai was 90. Abraham was pretty sure this was not going to happen. But God had different ideas:

> *Then God said to Abraham, "Regarding Sarai, your wife—her name will no longer be Sarai. From now on her name will be Sarah. And I will bless her and give you a son from her! Yes, I will bless her richly, and she will become the mother of many nations. Kings of nations will be among her descendants." Then Abraham bowed down to the ground, but he laughed to himself in disbelief. "How could I become a father at the age of 100?" he thought. "And how can Sarah have a baby when she is ninety years old?" So Abraham said to God, "May Ishmael live under your special blessing!" But God replied, "No—Sarah, your wife, will give birth to a son for you. You will name him Isaac, and I will confirm my covenant with him and his descendants as an everlasting covenant" (Genesis 17:15-19).*

Maybe you, like Abraham, are tempted to laugh—or cry—in unbelief concerning your infertility battle and God's ability to give you a child.   That's okay!

You and Your Faith Are Important to God

You matter to God. It's okay to be honest with God about your doubts and fears. God knows them anyway. Don't try to be a tough guy who doesn't waver in faith. Talk with God about any concerns. Listen for His wisdom and assurance. You are so important to Him. Your faith as a father-to-be is very important. This is not just your wife's issue.

God Wants to Cure You, Too

If you, like Abraham, need healing, know that God wants to heal you and make you fertile. Maybe you are older or maybe your sperm count is weak or slow or even nonexistent. God cares! This is nothing to be ashamed of. Get help if you want, but by all means, trust God for healing and know He is ready to bless you and your wife with a child. Don't allow a dire doctor's report to bring unbelief or cynicism to your heart. Have faith in the God of the Impossible. Talk to Him. Ask Him your questions. What a privilege it is to talk with God and ask Him for the help you need. Most "gods" demand sacrifices, but our God wants to bless you. He is pleased by your childlike dependence on Him. He wants to cure you, too.

> However, most guys are not the ones dealing with the physical problems of infertility. This gives the men a faith advantage that the women do not have. Men can ask in faith when women have doubts.

Praying for Your Wife

However, most guys are not the ones dealing with the physical problems of infertility. This gives the men a faith advantage that the women do not have. Men can ask in faith when women have doubts. While the women have to see the monthly menstruation that says once again they are not pregnant, or feel the excruciating pain of endometriosis, the men can more freely and easily exercise faith-filled prayer without distracting symptoms.

Men, model yourselves after Isaac, the miracle son of Abraham and Sarah. Isaac prayed for his wife, Rebekah, who, like many wives, was desperate after 20 years of infertility:

> *Isaac pleaded with the LORD on behalf of his wife, because she was unable to have children. The LORD answered Isaac's prayer, and Rebekah became pregnant with twins (Genesis 25:21).*

Watch out, guys! Earnest prayer may result in twins. But twins or no twins, prayer is powerful.

More importantly, unlike Isaac and Rebekah, we now live under the New Covenant. While it is still great for husbands to pray for wives, as Isaac did for Rebekah, now we can do this together. We are equal partners in this New Covenant life, though not all agree with this view. Let me explain.

Harmful Teaching

Some harmful teaching in the church about the husband-wife relationship puts unbiblical demands on the husband to "cover" or rule over his wife, who submissively depends on him for all. This puts a heavy burden on the husband that is really not his to carry. This was actually part of the curse in the Garden:

To the woman He said, "I will greatly multiply your pain in childbirth, In pain you will bring forth children; Yet your desire will be for your husband, And he will rule over you" (Genesis 3:16).

Now, under the New Covenant, sealed with the blood of Jesus, all are redeemed from this curse. Men and woman lovingly cooperate and are in partnership.

Equal Partners

Today, while men and women have obvious differences, they are equal partners in this new life in Christ. What a relief! Men do not have to have all the answers and be everything to their wives. Jesus has all the answers and He is a faithful Mediator for both men and women.

Women, isn't it liberating to partner with our husbands because Jesus is the Head of our homes? Men, isn't it a joy to share responsibilities for the family with your wife, knowing Jesus "covers" both of you? Together, we can treat one another honorably and always seek oneness and unity in our decisions as we mutually submit one to another. This is partnership at its finest!

Powerful Partnership Prayer

This cooperation brings such power to our marriage and to our prayers. My husband and I have experienced this over and over in our 45 years of marriage. And it changed our lives, not only as husband and wife, but also as father and mother. Peter wrote of this partnership:

In the same way, you husbands must give honor to your wives. Treat your wife with understanding as you live together. She may be weaker than you are, but she is your equal partner in God's gift of new life. Treat her as you should so your prayers will not be hindered (1 Peter 3:7).

Together, husbands and wives can pray about their infertility and the different nuances of their specific situation. Most of all, they can ask in faith for the child the Father is so ready to give and thank Him for the answer while they wait in peace. This will dispel worry and anxiety:

Don't worry about anything; instead, pray about everything. Tell God what you need, and thank him for all he has done. Then you will experience God's peace, which exceeds anything we can understand. His peace will guard your hearts and minds as you live in Christ Jesus (Philippians 4:6-7).

We can live this truth in all areas of our lives—health, finance, work, and family. We can tell God what we need. He will supply. It is His 100-percent guarantee to bring us the very things money itself can never buy. We can make daily thanksgiving and meditation on His Word a part of our routine. Then, our faith in God's unfailing love and faithfulness will grow strong and impenetrable.

Men Cannot Be God

Men may feel helpless, but they are not alone in this feeling. It is as old as the Bible. Jacob, one of the twins born to once-infertile Rebekah, felt very helpless when he, like his father, Isaac, had an infertile wife, Rachel:

> *When Rachel saw that she wasn't having any children for Jacob, she became jealous of her sister. She pleaded with Jacob, "Give me children, or I'll die!" Then Jacob became furious with Rachel. "Am I God?" he asked. "He's the one who has kept you from having children!" (Genesis 30:1-2).*

Maybe you have felt the pressure to somehow "be God" and miraculously empower your desperate wife to conceive. You feel helpless. Your helplessness ignites anger, and no one wins. Refuse to be like Jacob. Even though he felt helpless in himself, Jacob could have prayed for his wife. True, he was not God, but he knew God! However, it was Rachel who cried out to God and was heard:

> *Then God remembered Rachel, and God listened to her and opened her womb. She conceived and bore a son and said, "God has taken away my reproach." And she called his name Joseph, saying, "May the LORD ADD TO ME ANOTHER SON!" (GENESIS 30:22-24).*

God is waiting to hear your prayers. God is not asking you to be strong and helpful and fix the problem. He wants you and your wife to call out to Him. He hears and answers. Your partnership is sweet, secure, and strong.

Beware of Self Pity

Self-pity can sabotage cooperation. It is tempting for the husband to feel neglected while his wife is so consumed with getting pregnant. Men can learn from the mistake that Hannah's husband, Elkanah, made. Hannah wept and wept, unable to even eat, in despair over her inability to conceive a child. Her husband did not have a good response:

And Elkanah, her husband, said to her, "Hannah, why do you weep? And why do you not eat? And why is your heart sad? Am I not more to you than ten sons?" (1 Samuel 1:8).

It's a good idea to have a healthy conversation with each other to air despair and discouragement, but don't play the self-pity card. That's not helpful. Do you really want both of you in the ditch of despondency?

This is not demonstrating good active listening skills! Don't comfort your wife by focusing on you. To say, "Am I not more to you than 10 sons?" misses the point entirely. That is comparing apples to oranges. They are not the same. Your value as a husband is incomparable to that of a child that will be the fruit of both of your bodies. Each is equally valuable, but in a completely different category. It's a good idea to have a healthy conversation with each other to air despair and discouragement, but don't play the self-pity card. That's not helpful. Do you really want both of you in the ditch of despondency? Of course not! Pull her up and out. Hold her tight. Let her know how much you love her and are with her in this.

You are in This Together, So Cooperate

Together, you want a child. So, cooperate. Together, face the strains on your marriage and recommit to keep your eyes on Jesus, not on the circumstances. Trust the Holy Spirit to bring correction when things get out of balance. Be quick to say "I'm sorry" and to forgive each other. Especially do not let the sun go down on your anger:

> *Don't let the sun go down while you are still angry, for anger gives a foothold to the devil (Ephesians 4:26-27).*

Anger gives the enemy, Satan, entrance into your lives. That's the last thing you want as you wage war together to enjoy the breakthrough of God in your lives. You are about to become parents!

Face Your Fears

The thought of parenthood can send some willies down your spine. It is not unusual for the husband to be less enthusiastic than the wife about starting a family.

Whether it is fears about sharing love or the extra money or loss of free time, there are legitimate reasons to feel some hesitation. Make sure you engage in honest conversations about these concerns. Often, when we face our fears and talk about them, they lose their power over us, and we can plan joyfully for the exciting days ahead. Cooperation is so healthy and invigorates our faith.

Will I Be a Good Parent?

Will I be a good father? Will I be a good mother? This is a legitimate question, especially if your parents were less than healthy role models. However, even those who had good fathers and mothers might still struggle with insecurities and fears, given the complexities and pressures of today's culture. This is another area where you trust the God who lives in you by His Spirit to lead and empower you to be the best parents. Being the Almighty Father, He knows how to deal with all challenges of parenting! Plus, it always helps to be an active part of healthy church family where you can learn from older, wiser parents who have already navigated some rough waters. This saved Hap and me again and again. The family of God is such a rich resource and strong support. I have also listed some great parenting books in Appendix D.

It Was Worth It!

"It was definitely all worth it!" Andrew exclaimed with delight. He gently unfolded the soft pink blanket that surrounded his newborn daughter's cherub-like face as a giant smile covered his own. Today was Child Dedication Sunday, and Andrew and Kate let the tears stream down their cheeks as we all rejoiced over the safe arrival of Lily Louise. Andrew was indeed so much more than a sperm donor. The two years of agonizing endeavor were over. Yes, it was definitely worth it. He and Kate had worked to cooperate with one another on this journey toward God's cure for their infertility. He was now a delighted dad, she a glowing mother. And all the hard-learned lessons paid off. Two short years later, he and Kate welcomed their second child, Judah James.

So remember, partnership with one another and with God is important as you together move towards that day that you, like Andrew and Kate, will announce, "We're pregnant!"

Every couple is unique, and God will give different instructions to each one. Listen to the Holy Spirit's specific instructions for you as you wait.

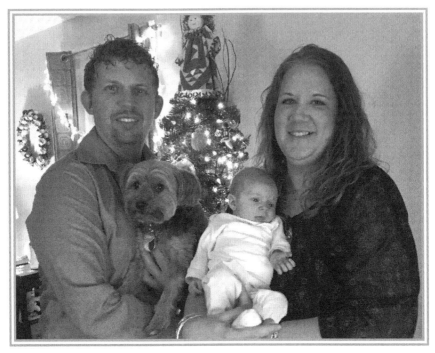

Shaun, Keri, and Kendall Greear

Partnering with God

Every couple is unique, and God will give different instructions to each one. Listen to the Holy Spirit's specific instructions for you as you wait. He may give you critical action steps to walk out your faith. He may emphasize prayers to pray together. This is partnering with God. He loves you, knows you, and is eager to see your family grow. But there is no formula! There is no "get pregnant quick" scheme. There is a God-given route to take, and He will be faithful to show you.

Radical Cooperation

Always ask the Holy Spirit for His unique instructions for you. For us, we sensed the Spirit instructing us to do some rather radical things. Please note we were following the Spirit's instructions for us. This is not a formula to follow. Our actions were following our faith in God and His word to us. I share ours as an example of how the Spirit worked in our lives to strengthen our faith and keep us giving glory to God. These were thoughts that came to our minds. We then talked them over, waited, and finally acted as we sensed this was God leading us to cooperate with Him.

No More Medical Treatment

First, I was to tell my local doctor that I would not be returning for any more care. I was to be clear that we were trusting God for a miracle baby. My doctor later told a friend of mine that I was crazy. (Okay, Jesus's brothers once thought He was crazy, too!) I would not return to my doctor's office until July 1978, a full 14 months later, and I requested a colleague instead of the doctor who called me crazy. Meanwhile, it truly was a refreshing decision to be done with all medical options for a season. For us, this was a wise move, because I easily depended too much on the doctor's skill and was quickly disheartened by any bad medical news.

If We Were Pregnant...

Next, my husband and I were challenged by the Spirit to think what changes we would make in our life right now if we were pregnant. Then, we were to begin implementing them. That was exciting! I bought some maternity clothes. I committed to healthy eating and exercising. We marked out the bedroom that would be the nursery. We compared prices of baby equipment. We pored over name books. Those were all fun activities. And, interestingly, they really did boost and strengthen our faith that God had heard and answered our prayer. We were having a baby. We needed to make some plans.

Now, I want to be clear that doing such things did not convince God of our faith, nor did it twist His arm or make Him give us a baby. That is foolish thinking, for sure. However, because those actions were a result of our faith in what God had done for us, they did reinforce our faith. It was a joy to cooperate with what God was telling us.

Crazy Cooperation

Then the Spirit told us to do something really crazy. This was a thousand times more difficult. Again, this came as a thought in our minds. We sensed God wanted us to start telling others that we were pregnant. What? That was going a little too far. That was downright stupid! Both my husband and I were in professional careers. Neither of us was given to grandiosity or exaggeration of any kind. But we knew we would not have come up with this outlandish instruction. We decided it must be God. We waited until we both felt at peace. This may sound a bit nebulous, but it simply means wait until you are both in agreement about a specific action. This may take some time.

Then, we chose to obey. Of course, we encountered a variety of reactions from people—both negative and positive. Those who were cheering us along on this faith journey were supportive and helpful. We had to choose to ignore the naysayers who knew we were not yet physically pregnant. We had to choose to not take the clucking of their tongues too personally or seriously. We knew we were cooperating with God.

Thankfulness!

Meanwhile, my husband and I thanked Jesus every day for our baby. We meditated on the promises of God from His Word. We revisited our prayer. Again, this is not asking again or begging God. We looked at the prayer we had written out and sometimes said it out loud again, more to ourselves than to God, because we believed we had received our answer already. But in repeating the prayer, we were reminded of the answer we had received, and it bolstered our faith. We were growing in our faith, sharing with others, and making choices to not look at the circumstances that often screamed our prayer was futile. All of these actions were done in cooperation with one another and with God. Sometimes it was easy and other times it was hard. But, always, we were thankful.

Results, But Not Instant!

We were married seven years, struggled with infertility for over three years, and waited 15 months for our specific prayer to be answered. But, God is so good, and cooperating with Him resulted in His cure for infertility and the gift of our first of five children.

> We all want instant results. Sometimes that happens. But most often your struggle with infertility is a journey. Now, though, you have some tools to move ahead. My desire is for you to have fresh faith that God has a cure for your infertility.

We all want instant results. Sometimes that happens. But most often your struggle with infertility is a journey. Now, though, you have some tools to move ahead. My desire is for you to have fresh faith that God has a cure for your infertility.

I encourage you to take some time and listen together for the next steps God has for you. Maybe you are ready to enter into a relationship with God for the first time. Maybe you are ready to ask the Holy Spirit to be more real to you and to fill you with His Presence. How might He be inviting you to partner with Him? Together, do what you think He tells you.   As you do, get ready to sing, "We're pregnant!"

Important Truths for Your Journey

* Your situation is unique and as such, your plan of action will vary from others' plans.
* God will show you how to partner with Him.

Suggested Action Steps

* Take inventory of your marriage and see where each of you may need to put some time and effort as you seek God's cure for your infertility.
* Ask God for any specific instructions for you as a couple.
* Read some resources that bring encouragement and help in areas of weakness.
* Do what God tells you!

Never Give Up!

"When doubts filled my mind, your comfort gave me renewed hope and cheer."
(Psalm 94:19)

As we conclude, if I could say just three words to you, they would be "Never give up!"

This can be a difficult choice when things do not change. It can be tempting to shut down your hope. Just last week I heard from a young couple who has been married for 11 years and had just about given up hope for a child. Now, they are 10 weeks pregnant and bursting with joy and thankful they did not give up. I want to encourage you to revisit the truths I have shared and allow hope to rise again.

God Wants to Give You Children

I trust by now you have seen that God wants to give you children. He is eager to cure you of infertility. He longs to remove any hindrances that prevent pregnancy. And He is ready to overflow you with faith in His love and power for you. He loves you and wants to bless you and multiply you. Recently, I was reading in my *One Year Bible* a familiar and powerful text:

And because you listen to these rules and keep and do them, the LORD *your God will keep with you the covenant and the steadfast love that He swore to your fathers. He will love you, bless you, and multiply you. He will also bless the fruit of your womb and the fruit of your ground, your grain and your wine and your oil, the increase of your herds and the young of your flock, in the land that He swore to your fathers to give you. You shall be blessed above all peoples. There shall not be male or female barren among you or among your livestock. And the* LORD *will take away from you all sickness, and none of the evil diseases of Egypt, which you knew . . . (Deuteronomy 7:12-15).*

This so captures much of what I have shared in this book. First, God loves you, blesses you, and wants to multiply you! Second, He blesses the fruit of your womb—the child growing within you. None will be barren or infertile. There is no fear of miscarriage. All sicknesses are gone. No evil diseases will come upon you. Good riddance PCOS, endometriosis, damaged tubes, low sperm count, hormonal imbalance, and unexplained infertility. Welcome healthy womb! Healthy mother and father! Healthy baby! If you are still battling with any of these issues, please try to not be discouraged and choose to trust God to show you steps to take to receive your healing and your healthy baby. Never give up!

Read Through the Lens of the New Covenant

Remember to read through the lens of the New Covenant and the grace of our good God. All these blessings are possible because Jesus died on the cross, defeated the enemy Satan, rose again, and now has all authority in earth and heaven. All sickness, sin, and death were laid on Him. He is the guarantee of a much better covenant than the one referenced above, where our strict obedience to the Law determined whether we received the blessings promised. Jesus fulfilled the Law. Jesus gave us His righteousness. Jesus sealed a new and better covenant with His blood. Trust Jesus, and you are included in this New Covenant. All conditions are met and blessings gush forth. These are promises to you. If you are unsure how to move forward, ask God.

Ask God for Wisdom

We have talked a lot about faith, prayer, healing, and removal of hindrances. However, you still might have some unanswered questions. I know how unique every couple and their situation is. I do not have all the answers by any means, but I know Someone who does—the All-Wise, All-Knowing God of the Universe who just happens to be your Father and invites you to ask when you need wisdom:

> *If any of you lacks wisdom, let him ask God, who gives generously to all without reproach, and it will be given him. But let him ask in faith, with no doubting, for the one who doubts is like a wave of the sea that is driven and tossed by the wind. For that person must not suppose that he will receive anything from the Lord; he is a double-minded man, unstable in all his ways (James 1:5-8).*

Know for certain God wants to speak to you about your unique situation. Know He gives generously to you. Know, too, how important it is to trust Him, to have faith that is strong and not wavering. I am sure God will impart to you the wisdom you need for your specific needs.

Listen for God's Voice

I urge you to get alone and talk to Him. Listen for thoughts that pop into your mind. Record these in a journal. Share them with your spouse or a close friend. Use this time to strengthen your relationship with Jesus, to be filled with the Holy Spirit, and to grow up into all God has for you.

Waiting is Hard but Helpful

Even though the pain of waiting is so incredibly difficult, God's timing is absolutely perfect for every situation. I am not minimizing the heartache that waiting often entails. But I can say with the utmost assurance, "in the fullness of time" you will bring forth your child. It will be the best time possible. Meanwhile, join with others who are waiting and support one another. Refuse to harbor jealousy or cynicism as you wait. Remember to be thankful that God has heard your cry and He is faithful to answer.

God Has a Good Future for You

None of us know the future. We can plan, predict, and try to control our destiny, but it is best to be still and know God is for you and He knows best. Choose to trust Him. Choose to rest in Him. Choose to enjoy today and know tomorrow is in His hands. Listen for His instructions. Obey with a joyful heart. Be assured that His love for you is unfailing. Know His faithfulness is unchanging. He has a good future for you.

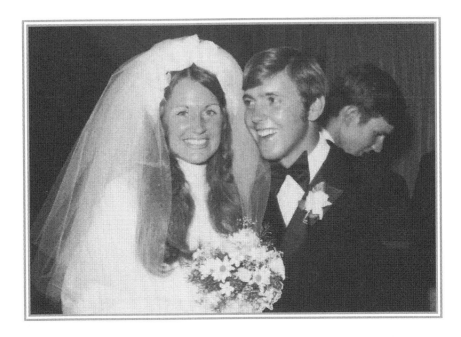

We Had Much to Learn

My husband and I had our future figured out. But we had much to learn. Like many young couples, we wanted instant pregnancy once we learned of the miracle-working power of God. We would have our baby, continue in our careers, and life would march on. However, we had to wait over 15 months before we knew we were pregnant. We conceived three months earlier but did not know.

While waiting, we started a Bible study in our home to tell others of Jesus and His mighty Spirit. During this time, we learned to study God's Word with the Holy Spirit as our Teacher. We learned how to pray in faith, thanking God for the answer we did not see or feel. We learned how to fix our eyes on Jesus, the author of our faith. We disciplined ourselves to get our eyes off ourselves and off our circumstances. We learned to be thankful and full of joy regardless of our present circumstance. We learned so very much that remains a part of our life today—almost 40 years later!

God's Plans Are Better Than Ours

All of this impacted us and radically changed the course of our life and our future. We faithfully met with others, prayed, shared God's Word, and waited. Over a year later, this small, home Bible study that we had started so we could discover more about God's miraculous love and power exploded when we shared our miracle pregnancy. Now, almost 40 years later, we continue to pastor that group of people. We multiplied into a large church where we proclaim and demonstrate every week that God is good and He is still doing miracles.

God truly knew what was best for our lives. He had a great future planned for us. We both left our careers and followed Him into a blessed, rich, and satisfying life. We rejoice that He made the infertile woman, me, the joyful mother of five children. We rejoice that He has made us, Happy and Dianne Leman, the exceedingly joyful (although sometimes exhausted) grandparents of 16 and counting. We also rejoice that we can share this story with you, pray for you, and be convinced that nothing is impossible with God. We are confident of God's desire for you to be fruitful and multiply.

Never Give Up!

You may be discouraged and tempted to give up. What good does that do? You are on a journey. God is walking with you. He will never leave you. Choose to keep going and growing. As I conclude this book, I want to answer some of the tough questions (Appendix A), share several more encouraging stories (Appendix B), give you some prayers to pray (Appendix C), and point you toward some helpful resources (Appendix D). All of these can strengthen you to not give up.

Stay in Touch

Please stay in touch through my Facebook page (**https://www.facebook.com/dianneleman1/**) or my website (**http://www.dianneleman.com/**) and share your good news of "We're pregnant!" so we can rejoice with you! Then pass on what you have learned, so others can know how to receive God's cure for infertility and they, too, will be singing, "We're pregnant!"

Appendices

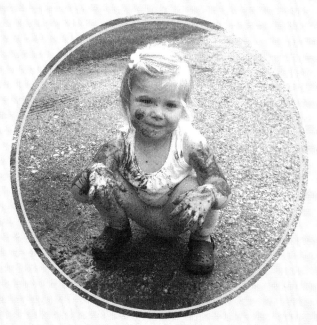

Emmery, daughter of Ed and Kara Moody

I know it can be oh so tempting to be discouraged, but my encouragement to you is "Never give up!" In these final pages, you will find many helpful resources, stories, prayers, and answers to your questions as you continue your journey to receiving God's cure for your infertility.

And, if you are still discouraged or have further questions, please visit my website at http://www.dianneleman.com/. I want to help you!

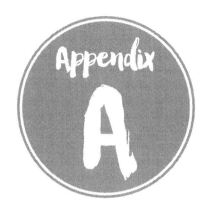

Real Answers to Tough Questions

When it comes to infertility, there is no end to the questions. They swirl like a gusty autumn wind through our minds and haunt us to know just a little bit more in hopes of finally getting what we so desperately want. With Google, we have such easy access to so much information. We can feel empowered by knowing. We can feel in control of our dilemma. However, answers alone, while temporarily calming, are no substitute for a vital, ongoing trust in the One who has all the answers. How incredibly honored we are to be called His children and to know Him as a loving Father who never changes and never plays favorites. He has all the answers and will share many answers with all who are in relationship with Him.

You Can Know God

If you have not yet entered into this amazing relationship with the Father through faith in Jesus Christ, please turn right now to Appendix C and pray the simple prayer of receiving His gift of a brand new life—eternal life. You can know God. Likewise, if you have never specifically invited the Holy Spirit to fill you to overflowing with His Presence, please go on to pray the next prayer in Appendix C for an infilling of the Holy Spirit. He is called our Helper, our Teacher, and the One who leads and guides us into all truth. He is God! He has so many gifts to give to enable us to live wisely and powerfully every day. He lives inside all of us who have placed our faith in Jesus. I often say we have the awesome privilege of having "Live-in Help," the Holy Spirit. He will lead you in discovering new truths and show you how to live in faith.

My Sincere Attempt to Answer Your Questions

Still, I know you will have questions. I don't have all the answers by any means, but here is my sincere attempt to answer what I consider the most common—and the toughest ones.

Questions About God

Why is this happening to me (us), God?

People often want to ask the "why" question, but I have not found that very help-ful. Instead, ask, "What does this mean?" and "What should we do?" Listen for His wisdom and be encouraged. Just remember, He loves you, does not play favorites, and wants to bless you with a child. Reread sections of this book that emphasize God's character and will—Chapters 3 and 4 especially.

I keep thinking (and several people have also told me) that God is pun-ishing me. Could this be true?

Absolutely NOT true! The glorious Good News is that Jesus took on Himself ALL your punishment for any and every sin you have and ever will commit. Believe Him and know that you are already 100 percent forgiven and clean in His sight. Of course, if you are continuing to willfully sin, you are denying the power of the Cross of Christ. Infertility is not a punishment from God. It is a medical condi-tion that often has roots in afflictions from Satan. (See Chapters 4 and 5.)

How can I know that having a child is God's will for us?

God's Word is very clear on this subject. Reread Chapters 2 and 4 and meditate on the Scriptures in Appendix D. He is the original Father. Family is His idea. "Be fruitful" is His first command. You can be assured this is His will—for you! Please do not base your faith (or fear!) on what has or has not happened for other couples. We don't know what goes on in the hearts and lives of others, but we do know God's Word and His character are true.

How can I know God better and hear His voice? I was raised without faith or in a faith that did not emphasize personally knowing God.

Being filled with the Holy Spirit is an absolute must for knowing God better and hearing His voice. (See Appendix C.) Because there are so many misconceptions about God, I would suggest you read *The Gospel in Ten Words* by Paul Ellis and *The Good and Beautiful God* by James B. Smith. These will give you a simple, clear explanation of the Gospel and God's character. I have listed several other resources in Appendix D to help you learn how to hear God's voice.

I noticed you interchange God, Father, Holy Spirit, and Jesus. I am confused! Do we have several Gods?

We have one God who is manifested in three Persons: Father, Son, and Holy Spirit. This is known as the Trinity. All three are coeternal, coequal. While each has different functions, They are still one and operate as a relational whole.

Several times I have seen prophecy mentioned as being helpful to couples. I thought this was predicting the future and is wrong for us to seek after. What is prophecy?

Prophecy as defined in the New Covenant is a gift of the Holy Spirit; it is mentioned in 1 Corinthians 12 and 14. It is God's words of encouragement, help, pictures, et cetera, spoken to another by an ordinary person. It sometimes has a future element to it, but most often brings comfort and faith to the person. You can learn more about prophecy by reading any of several books I list under prophecy in Appendix D.

Questions About Healing

How can I be sure of God's will to heal? It seems so many people are not healed.

In America, we are surrounded by the most advanced medical options and we are trained to depend on the expertise of doctors. So, it can be a switch to see God as a healer. Please read and reread the four Gospels—Matthew, Mark, Luke, and John—and let the Holy Spirit convince you that Jesus is a healer who is ready to heal you. I have also listed several good books on healing in Appendix C. *The Essential Guide to Healing* by Bill Johnson and Randy Clark is a very helpful resource, as is *Power Healing* by John Wimber.

I have prayed for healing and there is no change. What do I do now?

Please reread Chapters 6, 7, and 8, where I detail how we often have to wait to see the results of our prayers for healing. During this time, ask God for insight or changes that you need to make to cooperate with His healing process. There may be dietary changes, exercise, sleep, or emotional issues He wants to address. He may direct you to take a certain medication. The important thing: know God wants to heal you and is healing you. Receive your healing by faith and listen for God's instructions.

We really cannot think of any specific hindrance (Chapter 5). Will this stop our healing?

While we almost always encounter a hindrance with each couple, there have been times we have not. Do not try to dredge something up. We can all think of things that might possibly be hindrances, but we are looking for what the Holy Spirit highlights. Usually, this just "pops" in your head and it might even be a picture or a thought that you would never have considered. He will show you how to pray about it. Of course, we always pray for healing and the blessing of a child.

If I trust God for healing, does this mean I cannot also use medical treatments like drugs or surgery?

No. This is not an either/or situation. God has given doctors much wisdom and skill, and we are free to access medical healing. See below for more on the use of medical procedures.

There is so much pain and suffering in the world. How can I believe God wants to heal? It seems He is powerless at times.

Our Loving Father God is large and in charge, but He is not in micromanaging, control mode. Remember, there is another player on the field—Satan—who is the perpetrator of all evil, pain, and suffering. While He is a defeated enemy, he operates successfully when people believe his lies or choose to live in harmful ways. Free choice is still ours here on earth, and humans have a way of messing things up! While the Kingdom of God (Jesus's rule and reign) has come, it is not fully here until He returns in total power and Satan is dealt with forever. Now that you know these truths, you can begin to trust God for His healing in His time.

Questions on Faith

I do not seem to have any faith. I doubt and worry and have been so disappointed by my failure to get pregnant. How can I get faith?

God gladly gives faith to everyone, as He is the author of faith and the One who strengthens faith. He always answers the plea: help my unbelief! Meanwhile, remember that doubt and worry must be consciously refused. Of course, you will have the opportunity to doubt and worry every day. Just don't stay there. Fix your eyes on God and His Word. Read Chapter 7. Meditate on your chosen Scriptures (see Appendix D) and let faith be strengthened in your heart. Thank Jesus every day for the gift of a child.

I am unsure how to put action to my faith. I do not want to pretend or fake something that is not true. What should I do to show I have faith for my pregnancy?

Every person is different and must ask God for what fits her or him. However, remember, you are not trying to convince God you have faith. You are simply acting on the fact that He has heard your prayer and you are preparing for the answer to come to you at any moment. Read Chapters 7 and 8.

Should I risk trusting God in this? I am afraid if I do, and do not have a child, my faith will be shattered.

Faith is risky. But, thankfully, God is safe and faithful. He is the One who gives you faith and strengthens your faith. Remember, this is a relationship of trust in a loving Father. Even if you are disappointed, open your heart to God again.

Questions About Prayer

How can I strengthen my prayer life? It is weak.

I list a number of prayer texts/books in Appendix D. Let the truth of these soak in, and then just begin to talk with the Father. He is a good Father. He wants to give you good things. Start asking for small things. Watch the answers come. This is a conversation with the God who loves you through and through. Prayer is not a ritual or a game of getting it right.

Who should I get to pray for us?

You can just pray as a couple, but it is so helpful to have others pray with you. See Chapter 6 for more specifics on group or team prayer. Generally, trusted friends who have faith in a loving God who intervenes in our lives and heals us are the best. Stay away from well-meaning friends or even ministers who want to discourage you from radically believing God for healing and for a child. This will damage your faith.

My spouse is uncomfortable with prayer. What should I do?

As you know from reading this book, you can pray yourself. But why not use this time in your life to grow as a couple in faith? Be gentle with your spouse. Trust the Holy Spirit to open his heart. Try simple prayers together. It is not the elegance of your prayer that matters; it is your heart posture. God is eager to answer! Read Chapter 8 together.

Is there a specific prayer we should pray?

Pray for the desires of your heart, which I assume, is a child! No certain words needed. Just pour out your heart. Read Chapter 6.

Do you pray with a couple more than one time?

Yes, if about six or more months have passed and we have not seen the answer of healing and/or pregnancy, we gladly meet again to ask the Holy Spirit for further guidance in prayer.

Questions About Medical Intervention

At what point should we seek medical help?

Most medical research recommends seeking help for infertility if a couple has had one year of unprotected sex with no pregnancy. If you are older (35+), you may consider getting help sooner.

How far should we go with medical treatments?

This depends on your own judgment, finances, condition, and other personal considerations. I do caution couples to make wise choices and not be dazzled by all the possibilities. I also tell couples to be alert for when they are putting more faith in the doctor than they are in God. One way to know if this is happening is you experience overwhelming despair when you receive another negative medical report.

This shows you really trusted medication or surgery to heal. This does not discount the emotional letdown that comes with such a report, but beneath that, keeping you afloat is your faith in a good Father who wants to bless you with a child.

What about "drastic" measures such as IVF, donor eggs or sperm, surrogates, and womb implants?

All of these more radical procedures carry serious ethical considerations. Each couple must make sure they are at peace and their consciences are clear before proceeding with anything questionable. You will note in some of the stories I share that couples wrestled with the ethical implications and came to a conclusion that was agreeable to both. Never do anything that violates your conscience. Meet with your pastor or a trusted friend if you need counsel.

Is there ever a time to just stop all medical help and trust God alone?

Yes. I often counsel couples to "take a break from doctors" just to help them rethink and hear God for their specific needs. However, this is never advised to "show God how I trust Him"! He knows your heart, and if He tells you to stop, then stop—but don't stop to manipulate Him or convince Him!

Questions About Other "Help"

What about things such as acupuncture, chiropractic, hypnosis, Chinese medicine, or other more avant-garde help?

Again, each couple must make these decisions according to their own conscience and faith. Some have had good success with these approaches. As with medical help, you can subtly find yourself trusting more in these than in God. I know people have been helped by these practices, though.

Is it OK to use an ovulation test so we can be sure when to have sex?

There is nothing wrong with that! However, I have seen people rely too heavily on these and actually miss their true ovulation. I always say it is best to have lots and lots of sex and not be overly concerned with the exact time of month. I have seen many women get pregnant at the most unlikely time in their cycle.

Are there other things we should consider?

Nutrition, exercise, weight, and lifestyle choices are all important factors to attend to. Good information is available on various websites.

Questions on Hopelessness

I am seriously depressed and discouraged. Should I seek help?

There is no question that infertility can bring a plague of hopelessness and depression. I sincerely hope that reading these chapters will ignite hope in you. Read this book with other couples that are waiting. Pray for one another. Discuss the Scriptures. Rejoice as one by one, pregnancy happens.

And it is never wrong to get professional help. I caution against medication, though, as that usually means you will have to delay getting pregnant. Try lifestyle changes, and most of all, know the Holy Spirit is the great Comforter and wants to release new hope and joy in you.

How do I handle other people's "good advice" that just brings more despair?

The simple truth is we have the choice whether to let people's comments plummet us into another bout with despair or to present us with an opportunity to share our newfound faith in God's goodness. Make up your mind to just smile, thank them, and say you are excited for all God has for you.

Questions About Those Still Waiting

Do you know of couples who have received prayer and not been healed? If so, what is your counsel to them?

Yes, we still have couples that are waiting to get pregnant. Every couple is different, and we counsel according to their unique needs and situation. Relationship with God is very personal, and I do not know what goes on between another person and God. I always encourage each person that God loves them deeply, hears their cry, and has the best future ever for them. Listen to His voice, and He will give you the next step on your journey.

What about foster care or adoption?

I am in absolute favor of foster care and adoption! Just last month, I wrote a letter of recommendation for a couple that has decided to adopt. She is over 40 and they feel this is best for them. I rejoice with them! Another couple that is waiting told me they have found such joy and fulfillment in being foster parents and are in the process of adopting the infant they have fostered this past year. Again, I rejoice! God is for adoption, and He gives couples the heart for this.

Below is a story of an adoption blessing from God.

Kent and Liana Butcher

(Following is an email I received from Kent Butcher.)

On October 20, 1998, at the regional church gathering in Carlinville, you, Dianne, and Ed Loughran prayed for my wife and me to be able to have children. (I remember the date exactly because I spoke on the phone with my brother about his daughter who was born that very day.) Liana and I had been married for 12 years and had not been able to conceive. While praying for us, you quite confidently declared that we would be "holding our newborn baby a year from now." I distinctly remember you saying that because, quite frankly, I was a bit put out by the proclamation!

Anyhow, fast-forward to the fall of 1999. We did not conceive, but, probably sometime around the end of September 1999, I got a telephone call from a nurse in our congregation asking me if we "wanted a baby." A coworker of the nurse had just discovered—to her surprise, somehow—that she was eight months pregnant. The nurse from our congregation told her coworker about us, and the pregnant woman said, "I want them to have my baby." Long story short, on October 18, 1999, Benjamin Butcher was born. On the 19th, we brought our newborn son home from the hospital, just one day shy of the year you had said we would be holding our newborn. He is now a wonderful young man!

So, yes, consider adoption. Invite God into this process, as you will need miracles here, too.

Questions Are Good

It is good to ask questions. Some people think it is not good to question God, but I don't think that is true at all. God is not one bit bothered by your honest, heart-felt questions. You are in a relationship with Him. He loves you very much. He is such a good Father. He will give you answers—sometimes in the most unusual ways! He can "pop" things into your mind. He can speak to you through a book, His Word, a message at church, a dream, a prophetic word, or even a movie or TV show. And that doesn't even scratch the surface of how He can communicate with you. Always be listening for His voice. Discern what you hear and share with a trusted friend, minister, or counselor, if needed. Feel free to contact me personally with your questions. Visit my Facebook page at **https://www.facebook.com/diannelemam1/**.

Be Still and Know God Loves You!

Waiting in stillness is so hard. We live in a noisy, fast-paced culture. There is a sense that we need to be "doing something." There are many voices vying for our attention. Delight yourself in the Lord. Worship Him. Let Him love you. Refuse to fret or worry. Rest in faith. He will give you the desires of your heart.

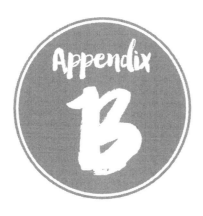

Miracle Stories

For this appendix, I contacted many different couples that received prayer and healing over the years and asked if they would be willing to write their stories. So many said "Yes!" I was truly overwhelmed. There are too many to share here. I know it is always fun to share such happy accounts of what God has done. I only include a few here to bring you encouragement. Don't let someone else's blessing provoke you to jealousy or self-pity. No! Let these stories remind you that God has a baby for you, too. He is still doing miracles. He is ready and willing to bless you, too. Under the New Covenant, it is so liberating to know that God does not play favorites! All who are His children through faith in Jesus can receive from Him. All of us can have our heart's desire. His favor is for you. He is waiting for you to receive His favor and blessing. Be encouraged and let faith rise in your heart as you read the stories of:

- Kara and Ed Moody
- Tim and Sarah Schiro
- Joel and Annika Smith
- Matt and Brittany Lappin
- Anita and Bas Hogendorf
- Katie and Jon Thorpe

- Isak and Hannah Im
- Laurice and Jonas Molina
- Judy and Dave Swartzendruber

The people themselves wrote the stories that follow; in some cases I have changed the names to protect people's privacy. I have only edited minor details. You will note how unique each situation is. Yet, God is the same loving, miracle-working Father to each one. He is that to you, too. Enjoy!

Kara and Ed Moody

Prayer had always been a big part of our lives, but the meaning of prayer changed for us on August 26, 2011. We received a phone call from our OB doctor notifying us that our pregnancy labs were decreasing and we were facing our third miscarriage. We were devastated. We had been praying for a healthy pregnancy and knew that it was God's desire for us, so why had we been through so much heartache? We began to doubt God and His promise. We knew that after a third miscarriage we would medically qualify to see a fertility specialist. It seemed like the right answer to help our heartache. We told our OB doctor to start the referral process.

Trust Me, I am the Ultimate Healer

As soon as we hung up the phone with our OB doctor we felt like God was speaking to us in a very intimate way! God kept telling us *Trust Me, I AM the Ultimate Healer, My desire is for you to have a healthy pregnancy.* So we hit our knees and began to pray! God knew the desire of our heart was to be parents, and we trusted that He would honor those desires! On Sunday morning we went to church, and during praise and worship, God was revealing Himself in a big way! We could sense the Holy Spirit's presence, and I got really warm and shaky and began to weep. I looked up at Ed and said we need to go forward for prayer and healing. As soon as the invitation was given to go forward we ran down to meet Di. We told Di that we had received news that our labs were indicating another miscarriage, but that we kept hearing God's voice through prayer that He was bigger than this. Di laid hands on us and professed that God's desire for us was to have a healthy pregnancy, and she prayed for healing over this pregnancy, future pregnancies, and my body. We left with confirmation that God was in charge.

That Wednesday I did miscarry. I remember thinking, *God, what was all that about? You spoke to us in a very real way. If You are the Ultimate Healer, why didn't You heal this?*

Through prayer, God just kept saying, *Trust Me. I am bigger than any fertility specialist. I am the Ultimate Healer of all things. I do know the desires of your heart, and I am faithful.* As hard as it was, we put our trust in His promise.

Pregnant?

A few weeks went by and I started having symptoms indicating I was pregnant. We thought there was no way. It was just two weeks prior that we had miscarried. But God kept speaking to our hearts, so we decided to take a pregnancy test and it turned positive immediately. We called our OB doctor to share the news and with hesitation she ordered pregnancy labs. Our labs were extremely high and kept climbing, a sign of a healthy pregnancy! We went in a couple of weeks later to see the beautiful site of our baby's heartbeat. We had conceived exactly two weeks after our third miscarriage—something that rarely happens, according to medical textbooks and statistics.

Thank You God!

Thank God He is bigger than any statistic, medical textbook, or fertility specialist. Thank You God for being so real, steadfast after our hearts, and faithful. God did prove that He is the Ultimate Healer! On June 2, 2012, at 7:09 a.m., the most beautiful creation, Emmery Katherine Moody, was born. Thank You, God, for answering our prayers.

Tim and Sarah Schiro

My name is Sarah and I was 23 years old when I married my high school sweetheart, Tim Schiro. He was only 20. Even though we were young, we both loved children and planned on starting a family right away. As the months passed without becoming pregnant, I became fearful that I would never become a mother and that it was my fault. In my teenage years I had struggled with life-controlling eating disorders that had affected my reproductive system and thyroid. Even though I was a healthy weight and had lived free of eating disorders since my teens, I wasn't getting pregnant.

Diagnosis of Infertility

When I was 25, I did receive a medical diagnosis of infertility. I was told this was common for women with my health history. Unfortunately, the treatment options available were not covered by our insurance. After prayer, my husband and I determined that we would pursue adoption through the foster care system instead of infertility treatment. This seemed like a good plan. After all, adoption had always been on our hearts for our family, but in my heart, I was devastated. I blamed myself for the infertility because of the eating disorders. I believed God wasn't answering my prayers for a child because He wanted me to understand the consequences of my sin.

This guilt and despair made it hard for me to pray or worship without weeping. I wanted to accept what I saw as the Lord's plan for our family, but I longed to carry a child in my own womb. My internal struggle broke Tim's heart. He believed that God was going to give us children through both birth and adoption.

Prayer

I grew up in the Vineyard Church and had heard Dianne's testimony of healing. I asked her to pray for us. As Tim and I prayed with the ministry team, I could see how the enemy was using my experience of infertility to cause me to question my fitness as a mother. I was so afraid that God wasn't giving me children because He did not think I was capable of being a loving, good mother. Also, though I believed healing was possible, I didn't think God would heal someone like me. I was afraid to hope and be disappointed, afraid of what unanswered prayers meant about my faith and my place in God's Kingdom.

As we prayed with the team, I felt the tight place inside me that had been filled with fear, shame, and doubt burst open. I was shaking and weeping, but I knew that the Holy Spirit was working inside me. Dianne saw a picture of Tim and me surrounded by children. We were laughing and filled with joy. I knew that picture was the family God had for us. We both love children so much and God was telling us that we would have children of our own. We chose to believe. After receiving prayer that morning, I committed to asking everyone we knew to pray for a miracle for us.

Help My Unbelief!

Over the next year my cycles became less regular than they had been before we prayed, and in the natural it seemed like things were moving in the wrong direction, but I became a prayer fanatic. I asked everyone to pray for us, and I prayed, too: *God I believe, help my unbelief.* When I was overwhelmed with the pain of infertility, I prayed over and over that God would "bless the pain." I didn't want the hurt inside my heart to destroy my faith in Him, but there were days when I felt like my faith was slipping away while I was waiting.

Sometimes I was angry because I felt like God was denying me what I wanted most in life—to be a mother. I knew He could heal me, but I doubted He would, and I told Him so. The blessing to this incredibly personal struggle with infertility was the transparency it caused in my relationship with God. I couldn't pretend that everything was okay. The pain of wanting a child stripped me bare before Him, and my prayers were more honest than they had ever been before.

God's Love

God loved me when I was angry, hurt, and doubting. I began to see His heart for me and to know that what was hurting me hurt Him too. I learned to contend in prayer. I knew that the enemy did not want me to be able to have children and that God wanted me to be healed. He wanted our home to be filled with the blessing of children and with joy. I began to pray in tongues during worship for the children I believed God was going to allow us to parent, both through birth and through adoption.

On Easter I was praying this way when I felt the Holy Spirit speak to my heart, "Sarah, I am giving you your children back from the dead." He showed me how the enemy wanted my future children dead and the physical deadness of my own reproductive system. I felt the Holy Spirit gently moving inside my body.

Pregnant, but Problems

Six weeks later, after another missed period, I decided to take a pregnancy test. It was positive, but even knowing how accurate the test normally is, I did not believe it. When the OB confirmed I was really pregnant, I was blown away. I told everyone right away and asked for prayers for a healthy pregnancy.

Around eight weeks into the pregnancy I began bleeding heavily. I prayed the entire way to the doctor's office. Once I was there, my doctor ordered an ultrasound to see if I had lost the baby. I kept reminding myself to trust God regardless of what the result was of this test as I watched the screen, praying to see a heartbeat. I knew that God was protecting the life of the child inside me, answering my prayers once again. Then I saw the flickering pulse of my son's heartbeat for the first time.

Our Gift from God!

Our son, Isaiah, was born on his due date, January 13, 2013, when I was 27 years old. His father and I know without a shadow of a doubt that Isaiah's life is a miraculous gift from God. When they heard the story of Isaiah's conception and birth, friends of ours began to share with us about their own struggles with infertility. We got to pray for them and see God touch their lives as well.

Tim describes us as miracle addicts, because we are at it again: praying and believing that God will allow us to conceive another child. God continues to surprise us with how good He is. I am not the perfect mother or wife. I still don't believe perfectly. I still get discouraged in prayer, but there are moments every day as I hold my son that I remember the miracle he is, and God reminds me that nothing is impossible for Him.

Another Miraculous Gift

Shortly after our son, Isaiah, turned one, Tim and I had a prophetic word about us having another baby, specifically a little girl. We began to pray in agreement with that word. After receiving the miracle of our son, we were full of faith that God had plans to expand our family. There were a couple times where we had thought I might be pregnant, only to find out I was not, but we refused to give up hope, because we sensed the Holy Spirit encouraging us to pray. We felt much more peace during this season of prayer and waiting. We were anticipating the good plans we knew God had in store for our family. Having both grown up close to our siblings, Tim and I did hope that Isaiah would have a sibling near in age to him. We prayed about that desire as well.

The day after Isaiah turned two we found out we were expecting again. On our sixth anniversary, our daughter Margaret was born. Her brother saw her minutes after she was born and serenaded the whole delivery room with a specially-prepared rendition of "I have the joy, joy, joy, joy down in my heart." It is so true. Our hearts are full of joy that God has given us these beautiful children and made us a family.

Joel and Annika Smith

We are Joel and Annika *(names changed)*, both in our late thirties. We struggled with infertility for nine years. There was no medical diagnosis for either of us, other than Joel had a low sperm count. However, we had a number of doctors tell us that it was still possible for us to get pregnant. There were no fertility issues on either side of our families, and we were both healthy adults. We tried artificial insemination (IUI) and it didn't work.

Ups and Downs

The struggle with infertility was never something I thought about having to go through. Unfortunately, for nine years it became the focal point of my life and faith. I had ups and downs. There were times when I searched the Scriptures and pressed in to hear from God about the battle we were fighting. Then, when more years passed and we still had not gotten pregnant, it all fell into question. My faith was strong at points when I found Scriptures to stand on, but again, when our dream never came true, it became harder to believe that standing on the Word was working. I do think that when you go through something like this for such a long time, you cannot escape the questions that come to mind about *why would God let this happen to me* and the like. When you find yourself with no sure answer to that question, it's a struggle to keep going.

Growing Spiritually in the Battle

One thing was certain, though. Just when I would get weary with one "approach" (meaning whether I was quoting the Word, listening to a specific ministry's messages, reading books, praying, etc.), God gave me something new—a different focus to inspire and encourage us in the waiting. We actually found ourselves growing a lot spiritually over the years, because we were searching for an answer to our battle. We learned things about the Word, the believer's authority, and the power of the Holy Spirit that we may have never encountered if we were not in such a desperate search. For example, we started learning more about the prophetic gifting and asked for prayer from various individuals, many of whom prophesied over us that we would have children, without even knowing our situation. This led us to seek and grow in understanding the gifts of the Spirit.

Fighting Depression

But on the other side of this growth was the deep emotional battle, and I struggled with trying to keep myself from being depressed. I thank God for my husband, because he was the only person in my life who really knew how hard this battle was for me, and he found ways to encourage me and keep us hopeful over all of those years. In addition, I quoted all of the "go-to" fertility and barrenness Scriptures and read the story of Hannah and Elizabeth many times in the Bible.

Prayer and Problems

We received prayer from the first year that we realized we were having fertility problems, so really, it was probably eight years of receiving prayer from anyone we could get to pray for us. One of the hardest things for me was watching literally all of my friends and family members have kids—even the ones who struggled with infertility and the ones who said they never wanted to have kids. Being an aunt to my nieces and nephews was difficult because it was a constant reminder of what I didn't have and didn't know if I ever would have.

On top of that was the struggle with watching some mothers mistreat their children or talk badly about their kids. I spent a lot of time praying and asking God for revelation about why so many young girls got pregnant when they didn't want to, and so many people had abortions. It was heartbreaking for me to think about it, but I felt like the answer God gave me was that His heart for all of His children is to have fullness and fruitfulness, even these young girls—His heart for them was to be a wonderful mother and raise amazing children. But, when people live their lives outside of walking with the Lord, they follow the world's path, and ultimately the same wisdom and support isn't there for them.

Seeking prophetically gifted people was helpful for us. While we were waiting, I did cling to the prophetic words that were given to us about children, even if they were given many years ago. Also, finding people to speak into your life who speak truth about the character of God, versus people who are trying to give you an answer for why you have to wait. It is so much more important to trust in who your Creator is than the possible reasons why you are not being given what your heart desires.

Question of IVF

Hopelessness was setting in after nine years. Do we or do we not pursue IVF? When we did finally start the in vitro fertilization process, I was still dealing with thoughts and beliefs about whether God would be in the process. The first week that we started with the medications, I prayed and asked the Lord for something to help me overcome that and know that He would be part of the process, and that morning I opened my Bible to this Scripture:

> All things were made through Him, and without Him nothing was made that was made (John 1:3).

This spoke to the fears in my heart, and I knew that if a child was created from the in vitro medical process, then it was still created by God. I was believing that any medical intervention in the process of creating a child was outside of God's hands and that if any of our embryos died in the process, we would be committing a terrible sin. There were different people in my life that had expressed this view, and I believed that I might be going outside of God's will and protection if I did in vitro.

When we started attending a Vineyard church in the Chicago area, the pastor shed a lot of light on these fears. He helped me see that, as God's precious and beloved child, He knows my heart is not to sin against Him, and He would not let us sin if we asked Him to keep us from that. I will never forget the conversation with our pastor where I experienced a revelation of this. His words to us were, "You're His kids, and He wouldn't let you sin if you ask him to protect you from that."

I can see this now in the Word; for example, the Lord's Prayer says *Do not lead us into temptation and deliver us from evil.* So, I trusted in God's love for me and my love for Him and asked Him this very prayer: if we did this in vitro process, don't let us do anything that would be sinning against You or outside of Your will.

Pregnancy!

I had a very good feeling when we were going through the in vitro process, and I won't say that I knew I was pregnant, but someone had given us a prophetic word before we started the process about a new and exciting season coming. So, that kept me hopeful in the waiting during the in vitro process. When the nurse from the fertility doctor's office called me, she left a message on my voicemail. I knew it was "the call," so I just got it over with and listened to it. I was overwhelmed with happiness at the moment I heard her say I was pregnant, and when I got in my car to go home that day I just cried and thanked God for His blessing. My husband and I went out to get Greek food (our favorite) that night and we called, texted, or Skyped all of our family members who knew we were waiting for an answer.

I will never forget my husband's 95-year-old Italian Catholic grandmother on Skype saying, "Annika, I told you God was going to give you a baby." And she really had said that for many years. Her faith is so simple, she doesn't know anything about "faith" or "prophecy" per se and has never read a Christian theology book in her life—she just believed that God was good and would give me a baby one day. I am so happy she got to see that day come to pass.

Trust in God, Not the Method

About five months into our pregnancy, we met another Christian couple who had undergone in vitro and only had one embryo to implant, which ended up not resulting in a pregnancy. They then became pregnant on their own many months later. As we talked with them about this, I was tempted to feel jealous that they had gotten pregnant without the in vitro process. But, then I realized that they still went through that difficult journey and the even more difficult part being that it didn't work for them.

During this conversation, I felt that the Holy Spirit gave me a revelation that I won't forget. We need to trust in the Lord God Almighty, and not in any particular method or process. I think this gets back to the Scripture about "fix your eyes on Jesus, the author and finisher of your faith," and the Scripture that says "My ways are not your ways and My thoughts are not your thoughts."

To someone struggling with infertility now, I would say, always put your faith in God's love for you and His good plan for you, not in anyone else's story, anyone else's success or failure, and not in any method or process. This doesn't mean you don't try different methods or processes in your hopes of having a family, it just means that everything is a means to the ultimate end of knowing God more intimately and trusting more and more in Him. I am definitely stronger on the other side of this. I feel less intimidated by others' opinions and less afraid that God will not provide for us in the big and small things of our life. I trust Him so much more than I ever did before we came through this journey. And, best of all, we were blessed with a perfect baby girl, Magdalena Grace.

Wisdom for Others

I would say that I have a stronger sense of trust that God is with me and that He has His hand in my life now. I knew this more on an intellectual level before, and now I feel like it is more settled in my heart. I still have a long way to go to being where I want to be in terms of faith and trust in Him, but overcoming the battle with infertility has given me a more solid place to stand in this.

What is the one thing I would like to say to couples who are struggling with infertility? Don't fear time and age—the God who created you and holds your life in His hands can give your body strength for anything He puts before you. Also, there is no "set" time or age for having children—just reading the Bible should tell you that.

So, don't fall into believing that as you get older it is going to get more hopeless or more difficult. I meet so many women now who have had children in their late thirties and forties. Other people's experiences do not have any bearing on your God-directed destiny, and the less you focus on other people and the more on God, the better off you will be in surviving this struggle.

Also, don't let anyone tell you that it isn't hard or you shouldn't be sad that you don't have kids. It *is* hard, and you have a right as a human being to feel sad, but do whatever you need to do to keep yourself out of depression and hopelessness.

Finally, enjoy your husband and work on your marriage as much as possible before you do get pregnant, because adding a baby to the equation is a whole new challenge for your relationship.

Epilogue

When my daughter Magdalena Grace was about 11 months old, we found out that I was pregnant with baby number two! We weren't even trying, and I was still breastfeeding. I wasn't on birth control since it wasn't needed for almost 10 years prior. God had other plans! So here we are, with another beautiful, healthy baby girl. Her name is Kia Marie, and she is perfect in every way. They are 19 months apart, so life is going to be crazy for a while! Rejoicing all the way!

Matt and Brittany Lappin

We are Matthew and Brittany Lappin, and we struggled with infertility for about three years. We are both in our late twenties. Ever since I, Brittany, was 13 years old, I was told by my doctor that I would never conceive. While seriously dating Matthew (my husband now), I made sure he knew of my "illness" and how the doctor said my only hope of having a child was to adopt. Though I am not sure he fully believed that it couldn't happen, I carried that weight until my husband and I moved to Champaign, Illinois. I was then diagnosed with PCOS at 23 years old. I was prescribed Metformin to help with the PCOS, but after taking one pill and becoming ill, we decided to wait until we made a future move to North Carolina before starting up again.

Learning God Heals

In Champaign-Urbana, Illinois, we got involved with a small group from The Vineyard Church of Central Illinois. They lifted us up in prayer. We heard messages on how God heals today and how He knows my heart and wants me to experience the joy of childbirth. It took a while for it to finally sink in but when it did, I could hardly handle my excitement. I was once afraid of God and doubted that He still healed. I thought that He had decided that I would not have a child, but I didn't know how to please Him or "talk Him into allowing me" to conceive. Never before had I been told that it was possible to conceive and have a healthy childbirth. I told everyone I knew. I was then able to pray for another couple in my small group at the time for infertility. Seeing their answered prayer after waiting for a longer time and experiencing more problems than I had, gave me a renewed hope.

Prayer and Scriptures

We received prayer from Dianne and her team on Mother's Day, one year and two months, before I conceived.

Scriptures that were helpful in strengthening our faith were:

Don't worry about anything; instead, pray about everything. Tell God what you need, and thank him for all he has done. Then you will experience God's peace, which exceeds anything we can understand. His peace will guard your hearts and minds as you live in Christ Jesus (Philippians 4:6-7).

Isaac prayed to the LORD on behalf of his wife, because she was barren; and the LORD answered him and Rebekah his wife conceived (Genesis 25:21).

It came about in due time, after Hannah had conceived, that she gave birth to a son; and she named him Samuel, saying, "Because I have asked him of the LORD" (1 Samuel 1:20).

Some Struggles

I began to have doubts and small bouts of depression. As much as I loved working in a daycare and loving on babies all day long, I longed to have my own. I loved to see baby dedications and rejoice with the parents when their children learned new things and experienced things for the first time, but my heart ached to be the proud parent. Holidays were especially hard. Seeing babies dressed in their Easter dresses or Christmas outfits, Happy Mother's Day written on all of my Facebook friends' walls. It was hard!

Support of Friends

Through it all, I had an amazing support system, people whom I could call and share what I was feeling, without condemnation, to be prayed for and loved on. Matt and I were so blessed to have people who stood beside us and boosted us at our low points. We gained new friends, a deeper relationship with our Father, prayer warriors, and a new understanding of prayer ministry and healing.

Meanwhile, we had friends who had dreams, visions, and prophecies for us. They saw my husband and me holding a child. While we were at conferences, people who didn't know us would come up to us and tell us that we were going to be parents.

Don't focus on all of the naysayers. I had plenty of people who tried to convince me to go on medicines, have surgeries, tell me that I must have sinned or

God would have blessed me by now. But, we never stopped trusting and believing that a healing was on its way. Focus on what God is saying to you. Put your trust in Him, and if He tells you to move across the country, move. Trust and follow what God has told you to do and He will be faithful.

New Home, New Baby!

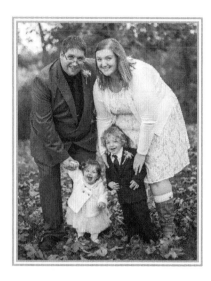

During the first week of living in our new home in North Carolina, I conceived. When I took the at-home pregnancy test, it was early in the morning and Matt was still in bed. I was so shocked to see two lines show up, I started yelling from the bathroom, 'Two lines, two lines!'" He awoke and as I walked into the bedroom he was crying and saying 'Two lines?" After showing him the stick we both we crying and jumping up and down yelling "Two lines!" It was one of the most joyous experiences I have ever had. We began telling others what He had done in our lives. Our healthy, bouncing boy, Arthur Lappin, was born April 16, 2015.

God Loves You

God loves you so much. He knows the desires of your heart. Allow Him to speak wisdom and comfort to you and hold those words close to you. Repeat them in the mirror. It helped me shrug off those who spoke ill to me.

The journey made me lean more on Him, trust Him, and have a deeper, more meaningful relationship based on love instead of the law. I have a freedom with Jesus that I had never experienced before this journey. I have true peace. The struggle is real, but it doesn't have to control you. Jesus spoke and calmed the storm. He will do the same with the storm in your life.

I would like to say a HUGE Thank You to everyone who prayed, supported and loved on Matt and me. You were there for us when it seemed like the world was against us. But, God is so good!! And.... we were pleasantly surprised with our second child Eleanor "Ellie" Marjorie just 4 months after having Arthur. Eleanor means "Shining light" and that is exactly what she is. She is such a happy loving baby. She doesn't know a stranger and greets everyone with a smile. We are so blessed to have her as a part of our family and our healing story.

Anila and Bas Hogendorf

My name is Anita, and I live in the Netherlands. I got married to Bas at the age of 22 in 1993. The first year we were okay with not having children, but after that it became a burden. We changed doctors and went together to meet our new doctor. He was nice and friendly and we told him about our wish to get pregnant. The next time I came alone to get checked. He was very rude and told me to stop feeling sorry for myself and get a life! I did not go back.

More Medical Stuff and Miscarriages

It took us some time before we went to another doctor. I was about 25 then, but she didn't take us seriously since she had spoken to the rude doctor. We had to fight to get through to a hospital. Our question was IF we could get pregnant.

They tested both my husband and me and did not find much that could stand in the way of pregnancy. I did have to lose some weight, my blood pressure was a little high, and my periods were irregular. Bas did not have very many active swimmers. But it was not impossible to get pregnant. I got medication for my blood pressure, and I had to make a curve of my periods and temperature. Bas had to start wearing loose underwear. Once my blood pressure was under control, they decided to give me Clomid medication to get a regular period.

I was pregnant the first time I took it but I miscarried. My doctor immediately put me on a higher dose and then, an even higher dose. I grew bigger and became aggressive and started to hallucinate. At that moment, Bas and I decided that it was not worth it. If God wanted to bless us, He would have another way. We said goodbye to the hospital. Sadly, I had three more miscarriages. But I knew we could get pregnant.

Lessons Learned

In the first years God spoke to me, saying, "It takes a village to raise a child." And He showed me how that had taken form in my life. That kept me on my feet for a long time. People told me many things. They all meant well, but I wanted to immigrate to the USA so I would not be faced with all those who did get pregnant. I was told over and over to pray Hannah's prayer. I refused! I did not want to bring my child to the temple, like Hannah did with Samuel. I wanted to raise my child myself. I did not want to settle for one child. I wanted a large family.

I believed that God would use everything in my life to a good purpose. We prayed and asked God for help. I prayed a lot on my own. I asked if there were things in my life I had to clean up. God showed me what was not good and He asked me to throw away a lot of things. At the time I did it because I wanted to obey. Now I know why. I had to throw away my novels because I used those to hide from real life. I had to throw away all my music that did not honor Him. Because singing is the language between God and me, I had to get rid of my many CDs that were not good.

The important thing here is, this was my journey. And I had to obey without expecting to get what I wanted in return! It was a hard lesson, but a great one.

There were times I did not want to pray about it. There were moments I could not pray. I felt very lonely. My husband was not there a lot of the time. He did not live on the same spiritual level. And people many times did not know what to say. But through it all, God was there!

What helped me the most was talking with those who understood me because they were going through the same thing or had been going through the same thing. Unfortunately, not many people were open about it. We decided to be very careful about who we told. Being honest without explanation turned out to be the best way to handle it towards the world around us. For example: "Yes, we want children; no, it's not going easy. Yes, we trust in God. No, I don't want to talk about it."

A Prophetic Prayer from the USA

Around the last part of 1997 we were planning to visit my friend in Champaign, Illinois. I wanted to move there and adopt children. In the fall we got a phone call on a Sunday from my friend. She told me that in her church that morning there was a call to the people from one of the elders that someone had a friend that was struggling with infertility. It took my friend a moment to realize that nobody else was raising his or her hand. So when Dianne repeated this, my friend raised her hand. And that morning, on the other side of the world, complete strangers prayed for us!

I thought it was funny. I did not know how to respond. As I came back in the kitchen where Bas and a friend were sitting at the dinner table, I told them what had happened. And the friend responded: "Anita, this is not funny. It is miraculous." Amazing! And at that moment it hit me! I was like Sarah. I, like her, lacked faith that I would have children of my own. I had started to make my own plans to immigrate and adopt. And I believed that it was God's plan for us. Though Bas, in his heart, did not really want that. He agreed more or less, actually less than more, just to make me happy and stop me from crying. I repented for that.

A Life-changing Visit

In the spring of 1998 we went to Champaign, Illinois. We had a wonderful time in the USA. We received lots of information about adoption. Bas got a job offer. I learned of an organization that would offer me a job right away. This job included a house and up to six children to care for. Finally, the day that we had to fly back to the Netherlands, just before we had to leave, we met Dianne at the Vineyard Church. She asked if I believed in God. She asked if I believed that Jesus died and rose again for my sins and if I believed in the power of the Holy Spirit. All three I answered with a yes! She asked the Holy Spirit to show us any hindrance. A picture of frogs came to my mind. I wasn't sure what that had to do with this. She told me a story about frogs and the Bible and infertility. And pretty soon I knew in my heart, I had to throw away my very large collection of frogs in any form. And when I got home, I did. When she finished she said, "Go home. Pray daily for strong faith, and trust in God."

Am I Healed?

When we came home I had my period right on time. This was a miracle. We were so happy to be healed in that part. The next month, I again had my period. The third month I did not get my period. Immediately, I became like Sarah. I cried! I did not think I was healed because I was not getting pregnant. Then Bas said to me that I should stop crying. "You might be pregnant. You can't stay away from that one brand of licorice." We did not go to church that day, but searched for courage to do a test. The test was positive. That Thursday we saw our gynecologist and we went home with a picture of a dot. Our baby was six weeks and five days.

Joep was born February 17, 1999. After a very difficult labor and delivery, they laid Joep on my belly. Suddenly, I saw a blue little face. I screamed that he was not breathing. They took him away and started to help him breathe. I prayed fervently for his life. Joep has been diagnosed with a rare form of autism, but he is doing very well! Today we have a healthy handsome teenager!

Surprise Blessings

Due to my traumatic pregnancy, labor, and delivery, I was told not to get pregnant again within the next two years. Based on my history, I thought it would take about five years to get pregnant. So when Joep was six old months, we stopped being careful about birth control. On July 5, 2000, just 17 months after Joep was born, our second son, Stijn, was born six weeks early. He struggled with some developmental delays and it was a difficult time for me with two small children. By the time we felt ready to have more children, it was 2003. My friend from

Champaign was over to visit her in-laws, and I told her in church I was pregnant. The next day it was my 33rd birthday, and I miscarried. But, the next month I was pregnant again. On November 11, 2004, our son Flip was born through an emergency C-section.

Around 2007, we found out about the autism, and because I was 38, we decided to be happy with the three wonderful blessings we had.

My Encouragement to You

Whatever your situation is, don't think that you will get healed and blessed with a child because you do the right things or believe in a certain way. Don't think that you are not good enough or don't believe good enough. Don't listen to people. Listen to God. Live your life with Him, for Him, and through Him. He has planned you before He made the earth. He put wonderful things in His plan for you. He holds you in His hand. Seek His will for your life. Trust in Him always. And when you find you can't believe, simply ask Him to forgive your unbelief and for Him to meet you in your unbelief. He is a God who answers our prayers and attends to our needs.

Katie and Jon Thorpe

Jon and I tried to get pregnant for about three years. Early on in our journey, we conceived naturally. We were ecstatic. Unfortunately, that pregnancy ended in a miscarriage during the first trimester. We were devastated and argued with God: *Why?* We tried to conceive on our own again, and we were not able to get pregnant. We decided it was time to pursue fertility treatments. Month after month, we discovered we were not pregnant. We were again devastated and argued with God, *Why?* I battled doubt and fear of not having a baby.

Hearing from God

Having quiet time with Jesus and journaling what I heard Him speak to me helped me the most. Know that God will fulfill the desires of your heart. One night when I was praying, God gave me a series of visions. Father God took me by the hand and led me to a hill that overlooked a field of apple trees (an orchard). After my vision, I looked up the meaning of an apple orchard: fruitfulness. I was encouraged, and I recognized that God knew the desires of my heart.

I was in constant prayer the entire time we tried to conceive. Worship music was also so helpful. I have a 35-minute commute to work, and I often listen to Christian radio stations. There were quite a few songs that ministered to me during my hard times of waiting. It was so frustrating, too, watching family and friends get pregnant. God gave me this Scripture from Proverbs:

> A heart at peace brings life to the body, but envy rots the bones (Proverbs 14:30).

He also highlighted other Scriptures that strengthened my faith, including this one:

> In the same way the Spirit helps us in our weakness. We do not know what we ought to pray for, but the Spirit Himself intercedes for us with groans that words cannot express. And He who searches our hearts knows the mind of the spirit, because the Spirit intercedes for the saints in accordance with God's will (Romans 8:26-27).

Trust Me, Katie, Not Medicine

Our next step in fertility treatments was in vitro fertilization. At that time, we heard very clearly from God: *Stop. I want you to trust Me, Katie. Not Western medicine or Chinese medicine. I am the Ultimate Provider.* We decided to take a few months off and work on our relationship and ourselves. I couldn't believe how straining this had all been on our marriage. During that time, adoption fell heavy on my heart. Jon is adopted and I have always thought about adoption. We decided to pursue international adoption through the country of Haiti. We found an orphanage and an adoption agency. After gathering the necessary information, we had all we needed to move forward with an international adoption. At that time, I, again, heard the Lord say, *Stop.* I was confused. I asked God for something to let me know what we were supposed to do. He gave me this Bible verse:

> For this child I prayed and the Lord granted me my petition, which I asked of him (1 Samuel 1:27).

Pregnant!

Jon and I decided to put off pursing the adoption process until summer, when we had more time to invest. Two weeks later, I found out I was pregnant, NATURALLY.

I can truly say I was shocked to find out I was pregnant because we weren't "trying." I was cautious the first trimester because my last pregnancy resulted in a miscarriage in the first trimester. How thankful we were to welcome our healthy son, Jacob Jonathan Thorpe, on November 11, 2013.

My Encouragement to You

My struggles with infertility, no doubt, brought me closer to Jesus. I know that He planned for us to be Jacob's parents in His timing, not ours. One thing Jon and I learned through our struggles was to "let go, and let God." It seems as though the second we stopped striving to achieve our goal of pregnancy, Jesus granted us the desires of our heart (a baby!). I realized God does not owe me anything, not a baby, not even an explanation of His choices. God sees the big picture, from the beginning to the end. I can only see my little piece right now.

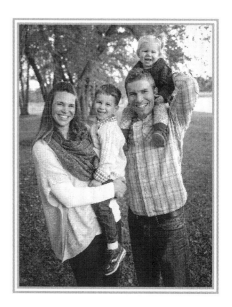

Surprise! When Jacob was 10 months old I found out I was pregnant. Our sweet daughter Julia joined us in 2015.

Isak and Hannah Im

We are Isak and Hannah Im from Korea. We came to the US from Korea in 2010 to do my (Isak's) postdoc course at the University of Illinois in Champaign-Urbana. We struggled with infertility for four years and eight months. But we had no known medical problems. Doctors said that they couldn't find any medical issues to our having a baby.

Journey Begins

We thought that God would give us children "someday." It was not like solid faith. It was a somewhat self-comforting idea while we had no answer. As time went by, doubt and fear that what if God doesn't give us a child arose in our heart. Sometimes, we thought that because of our sin and shortcoming, God is training or punishing us.

Then we started to read books of various authors from the "faith movement" and the Pentecostal movement, which are new to us. We were excited to find out "hidden" biblical truths about healing and other supernatural gifts of the Holy Spirit. Then we attended some healing meetings to see some evidence. Our faith about healing has grown continually as we participated in more meetings and experienced real healings of our own and others. We started attending the Vineyard church in Urbana, Illinois, to pursue this work of God, because our former church was not open to that and we had some conflict.

Waiting Time and Medical Help

In summer 2011, we received healing ministry for the first time in Chicago from a pastor from Korea. When we received prayer at the healing meeting, my wife experienced several healings such as back pain, one shorter leg growth, cold hands and feet. She felt some warmth at her womb when she received prayer as well. There was no sign of pregnancy for about one year since we had followed this supernatural healing secretly. It had been three years since we'd been married at that time. My parents wanted us to get some help from the hospital and we decided to do in vitro fertilization. So Hannah went back to Korea to receive the IVF procedure, and I remained in the US, because our health insurance in the US didn't cover the IVF.

There was a good sign of success at the beginning, but it failed because there was no heartbeat. We were very sad and frustrated. Hannah came back to Champaign with a wounded heart and body. All the effort and money we had spent for six months resulted in failure and disappointment.

Prayer and Community

While Hannah was gone, I joined the Vineyard church in Urbana and attended a small group. Our small group members prayed for Hannah while she was in Korea. When Hannah came back, our small group leaders, Steve and Ana Price, introduced us to Dianne to receive prayer for infertility on 8/12/2012. It was a very good meeting. We felt loved by Dianne and other members who attended the meeting.

Although we tried many things, including natural and supernatural things, we didn't receive an answer. But our heart became closer to God. Our faith in healing became stronger. We didn't give up, and requested prayers and received prayer when we had the opportunity. As we sought God's presence and the work of the Holy Spirit, infertility was not really a problem in our life. We were happy to see what we couldn't see before. We were happy to know the truth that we didn't know before. And fellowship with the people following the same faith really helped us and cured our hurt. It was really encouraging and helpful when we had a community of the same faith.

Prophecy

We traveled to Washington, DC (October 2012) to attend a meeting held by a Korean church group. It was a small meeting, and we had a group training time about prophecy. One guy from Korea who is a total stranger to us gave me (Isak) a prophecy. At the end of his prophecy he mentioned that he saw a picture of a sonogram. He felt that its meaning was more in the physical realm than the spiritual realm. He said that God wanted to give us a child as a gift. That was really encouraging because he didn't know our family situation.

Then we returned to Champaign. At our small group meeting that week, some of our members felt some special heart for our family's baby issue and prayed for us. Ana Price shared something like "the time has come and you are ready'" (I don't exactly remember). Then I remembered that Josh, who plays guitar at the Vineyard, gave me a prophecy about the blessing of a child to my family on Sunday morning ministry time the week before we went to DC.

Perfect Timing

That week was the perfect timing. That week was also the only available week for us to have a baby. We knew it was God who planned this. We couldn't deny that God was working behind this. So, two weeks later, we did a pregnancy test. It was positive! A few weeks later a doctor confirmed it. Our healthy, handsome son, Daniel, was born on June 29, 2013. We are so thankful!

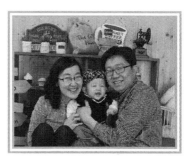

Laurice and Jonas Molina

Jonas and I had been married five years and tried for three years to get pregnant. We never formally sought medical input, since we believed that we would eventually conceive. (Even though so many days we struggled to believe!) For three years we were fortunate to have been prayed for by others. Several people gave us some prophecies that strengthened our resolve to wait upon the Lord. The Lord has been so near to us, so even through negative after negative pregnancy test. He would just comfort us and dry our tears.

Study God's Word

It was during this time as well that I just dug deeper into the Word. I was given a fresh desire not just to study His Word but to live it out and pray out the Scriptures that the Father highlighted to me. I felt a new boldness to share about my struggles, and still have the passion to pray for people as my prayers have yet to be answered. In my daily talk with Jesus, I have felt in my heart His audible voice and His expressions of just how much He loves me and how He delights in giving me the Kingdom. He has lifted my weary head and worn-out faith by providing me friends who breathe words of encouragement to me and lovingly pray for Jonas and me. I found myself wanting to open my home to small group meetings and also looking forward to our alone times with the Father. Many times, Jonas and I went to our knees together in prayer as the waiting took a toll on us.

Meaningful Scriptures in My Journal

As I look through my journal, my heart warms as I remember the many Scriptures that held my faith walk together:

> *"Then Abraham waited patiently and he received what God had promised."*

The wait really grew my character; it humbled me because I used to be so proud about being patient. But Jesus gently rebuked my prideful heart. He taught me patience, like how He is, and not how I think I should be. Truly, His ways are not my ways, and His thoughts are higher than my thoughts.

> *'Therefore, we who have fled to Him for refuge can have great confidence as we hold on to the hope that lies before us."*

How amazing it is to be constantly reminded that as daughters of the Most High God, we are never without hope. Even if tomorrow looks bleak, we have a Father who is not fazed by our circumstance. I just love that about Him. I can be myself in the arms of my Father—angry, bitter, questioning, and doubtful, and not once have I felt that He has shunned me because of my attitude.

> *'The Hope is a strong and trustworthy anchor for our souls. It leads us through the curtain into God's inner sanctuary."*

I now look at this, in hindsight, as something that really made God reveal another facet of His Lordship—there is so much more to Him that I have yet to know. I am speechless by what I have known about Him so far, yet He keeps on revealing Himself, glory after glory.

"When I pray, You answer me and encourage me by giving me the strength that I need."

The thing with the Father is, not only does He care about my desire to have a baby; He cares about the whole picture. So many times our marriage was strengthened when we felt especially doubtful that we were even going to conceive. Scriptures were just highlighted, friends called and gave us encouragement, or we found that Jesus was personally talking to us separately, to lift each other's spirits. God is so personal! We have felt His profound hand cradling our hearts.

"Pray diligently . . . with your eyes wide open in gratitude."

I started to journal at a very young age, and it was during this time of waiting that I felt compelled to look back and read my older entries. To reminisce on the faithfulness of my Father brought many tears. His track record in my life has always been stellar. He has never failed me. He delights in me and He always fills me with good things. In the mornings when I sit on my big couch and I bawl in His presence, He lovingly directs my heart posture to one of gratefulness, and it shifts my focus on the things that He never held back from me—His very self.

"As each one has received a gift, minister it to one another, as good stewards of the manifold grace of God."

We have experienced firsthand the gifts of prophecy and countless blessings prayed over us from our small group, our prayer leaders and pastors, and even complete strangers. Somehow in the three years of our waiting time, the boldness in our hearts increased to also do the same for others. I personally feel this tugging feeling as Jesus pours into me the gift of discernment and words of prophecy for me to give to random people I meet every day.

I also realized my experiencing unanswered prayer is not a hindrance for me to pray for other women who are going through the same thing. The experience has opened my eyes to see that there were a lot of us going through that, and how appropriate it is for me to pray for them! I think Jesus made sure that these other women also get the encouragement they need to hold on to the HOPE that I have experienced!

"And I will give you a new heart with new and right desires, and I will put a new spirit in you, I will take out your stony heart of sin and give you a new, obedient heart."

A funny thing happened during this time. While I started painfully aching for a baby to warm my arms, in the long run of the wait, my heart shifted to a fresh desire to seek my Father, to "taste and see" who He is, and not run after Him for the "stuff" He can bless me with. I responded to His call to really get to know Him more profoundly and be more cognizant of who He is to me. Our talks early in the morning can be quiet and uneventful, or they can be loud and wild with worship music. He meets me where I am.

Pregnant!

We found out I was pregnant shortly after we celebrated our fourth anniversary. What an amazing time of preparation it was for us, filled with highest of highs and lowest of lows. The faithfulness of the Father has never been so highlighted! In my heart I really do believe I relearned how to be His daughter so I may be the best parent. I gave birth to Jade Louise on October 27, 2013. We know how to "point her to the way she should go." Our resolve is to introduce her to Jesus, the Lover of her soul.

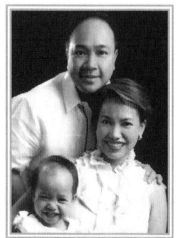

"I have no greater joy than this, to hear of my children walking in the truth."

I have started praying this when Jade was still in my womb. She has been skillfully and wonderfully made. I praise the hands who have molded her, her personality, her heart, her desires. I worship the One who has loved her before she came to be. So many times I am caught off guard just feeling so much love and compassion for this helpless infant in my arms, and sensing the Holy Spirit tell me, "That's what I feel about you." I also know deep in my heart that how He loves is so much more than how I can ever love my daughter. Oh, how the Father equipped us with Himself, that we may parent how He parents us.

Judy and Dave Swartzendruber

In August 1982, the Holy Spirit convicted my husband, David, that perhaps it wasn't the Lord's will that he had had that vasectomy over five years before. Maybe God wanted us to have more than our two boys we had, 21 and 20 years old at that time.

David repented and asked forgiveness for not having even made the vasectomy a matter of prayer. Together we prayed that the Lord would have charge of the size of our family. We didn't pray for more children; we just gave that decision to God.

I missed my early October menstrual period, and on October 30, my pregnancy test results were positive. We were so excited!

Decisions

Our boys both had their own homes. We had an empty nest. I was 41 years old and David was 44. It was exciting to tell our family and friends that we were experiencing this miracle from God. Here we were, really expecting just one month after we had prayed together. We faced a major decision about my prenatal care. Because of my age and the fact that our first son was born by C-section, I knew that I would be considered "high risk" by the medical profession. We knew that this was God's miracle and asked ourselves, "Why would God give us this baby if it was going to cause me or the baby any problems?" We had great peace to trust Jesus for a perfect pregnancy and childbirth, and to us that meant not going to an OB doctor. We really had a knowing that this was what God wanted us to do. Thus we began this journey with Jesus as our Doctor. We prayerfully sought guidance during the pregnancy and ordered a home birthing supply kit.

Defining Prayers

We had three defining prayers: first, I wanted to shop, so I wanted to know if we were going to have a boy or a girl. God showed us that our baby was a girl, so I filled the closet with little girl baby clothes and decorated the nursery with peach and turquoise flower prints.

Our next prayer was for her name. We knew God would want a special name for her. He told us her names should be Sarah (since we were older) and Joanna from Luke 8:3.

The third prayer was very important to us. "When, Lord, is she going to be born?" David was driving to Chicago five nights a week for UPS, and I knew he couldn't be out there at work when the baby was coming. We prayed separately and we each had the date of June 16, 1983.

Giving Birth

We had to stay positive and in faith, and it was a wonderfully exciting time. I had a healthy pregnancy, especially considering that I was now 42.

On June 15, 1982, David finalized his vacation schedule so that he would be at home for the birth the next day. The first contraction came about 8:15 a.m. the following morning. I worked around the house, "nesting," fixing food, cleaning, getting the baby clothes out, and setting up the home birthing kit. About 4:30 in the afternoon, I couldn't walk through the contractions anymore, so I lay down. Sarah Joanna was born at 7:44, weighing eight pounds, eight ounces. What a wonderful experience! We played praise music during the evening. It was a peaceful, pain-free delivery. She responded right away and was a normal healthy baby as well as a healthy, happy, and peaceful girl as she grew up.

She is a blessing. This awesome experience of God's miraculous love and power changing our lives and family circumstances forever has caused us to grow in our relationship with Jesus and to trust Him more in every situation of life, no matter how impossible.

Note from Di: *I am privileged to hear new stories every month and am always so thankful that God continues to bless couples with the precious gift of a baby. I keep a list in my journal of couples I am praying for to get pregnant. It was such a joy at the close of 2016, just as this book is getting ready to be published, to note that seven more couples are pregnant or recently gave birth. Please visit my website to read new stories and please send me your story so we can rejoice with you.*

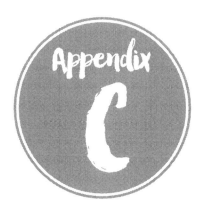

Prayers for Your Journey

Prayer is simply talking with God. We can make it so complicated. Of course, the most important prayer is receiving Jesus as your Savior, followed by the prayer for the infilling of the Holy Spirit. The other prayers are just examples of how to pray about these specific topics. I encourage you to write your own prayers, using Scriptures that are meaningful to you and concerns that are unique to you.

Prayer to Receive Jesus as Savior

Jesus, I want to receive you as my Savior, my Lord. I turn from my old thoughts and behaviors and ask you to take over my life and make me new. I believe You died for my sins, You were buried, and You rose again. Thank you that all my sins are forgiven and gone! Thank you that I have a new heart and new life, now and forever. I love you, Jesus.

Here are helpful Bible texts on becoming a new person in Jesus:

But to all who did receive him, who believed in his name, he gave the right to become children of God, who were born, not of blood nor of the will of the flesh nor of the will of man, but of God (John 1:12-13).

And I will give you a new heart, and a new spirit I will put within you. And I will remove the heart of stone from your flesh and give you a heart of flesh. And I will put my Spirit within you, and cause you to walk in my statutes and be careful to obey my rules (Ezekiel 36:26-27).

If you confess with your mouth that Jesus is Lord and believe in your heart that God raised him from the dead, you will be saved. For with the heart one believes and is justified, and with the mouth one confesses and is saved. For the Scripture says, "Everyone who believes in him will not be put to shame" (Romans 10:0-11).

For God so loved the world, that he gave his only Son, that whoever believes in him should not perish but have eternal life. For God did not send his Son into the world to condemn the world, but in order that the world might be saved through him (John 3:16-17).

Prayer for Infilling (Baptism) of the Holy Spirit

Jesus, I thank you for your Holy Spirit. I want to overflow with your Spirit. Please fill me and empower me to live and minister like You. Please fill me with all of Your gifts.

(If you want to receive the gift of tongues or speaking in an unknown language, just open your mouth and begin to speak, but not in your native language.)

Helpful verses:

On the last day of the feast, the great day, Jesus stood up and cried out, "If anyone thirsts, let him come to me and drink. Whoever believes in me, as the Scripture has said, 'Out of his heart will flow rivers of living water.'" Now this he said about the Spirit, whom those who believed in him were to receive, for as yet the Spirit had not been given, because Jesus was not yet glorified (John 7:37-39).

For John baptized with water, but you will be baptized with the Holy Spirit not many days from now . . . But you will receive power when the Holy Spirit has come upon you, and you will be my witnesses in Jerusalem and in all Judea and Samaria, and to the end of the earth (Acts 1:5-8).

And he said to them, "Did you receive the Holy Spirit when you believed?" And they said, "No, we have not even heard that there is a Holy Spirit." And he said, "Into what then were you baptized?" They said, "Into John's baptism." And Paul said, "John baptized with the baptism of repentance, telling the people to believe in the one who was to come after him, that is, Jesus." On hearing this, they were baptized in the name of the Lord Jesus. And when Paul had laid his hands on them, the Holy Spirit came on them, and they began speaking in tongues and prophesying (Acts 19:2-6).

I'm grateful to God for the gift of praying in tongues that he gives us for praising him, which leads to wonderful intimacies we enjoy with him. I enter into this as much or more than any of you. But when I'm in a church assembled for worship, I'd rather say five words that everyone can understand and learn from than say ten thousand that sound to others like gibberish (I Corinthians 14:18-19 MSG)

If you have more questions, see Appendix D for books on the Holy Spirit.

Prayers Concerning Conception, Pregnancy, and Childbirth

I like to use Scriptures when I pray, because it is a clear revelation of God's will. This gives us confidence that God hears and answers our prayer:

And this is the confidence that we have toward him, that if we ask anything according to his will he hears us. And if we know that he hears us in whatever we ask, we know that we have the requests that we have asked of him (1 John 5:14-15).

As a couple, use Scriptures that are meaningful to you and rewrite the following prayers. Also, check out some of the books in Appendix D for more samples of prayers, especially under the *Childbirth* section.

Prayer to Receive a Child

Father, we thank You that it is Your will to bless us with a child. We ask in Jesus's Name for the perfect conception of the child You have for us. We believe You want to give us a child and we receive this gift.

A few helpful verses:

He gives the barren woman a home, making her the joyous mother of children. Praise the LORD! (Psalm 113:9).

Behold, children are a heritage from the LORD, the fruit of the womb a reward (Psalm 127:3).

Prayer for a Healthy Baby

Father, we ask You for a 100-percent healthy child, perfectly formed in my womb. We ask this because we believe You are the Giver of Life and the Great Physician. We know You are fearfully and wonderfully developing our baby. Thank You in Jesus's Name.

Some verses to meditate on:

For you formed my inward parts; you knitted me together in my mother's womb. I praise you, for I am fearfully and wonderfully made. Wonderful are your works; my soul knows it very well. My frame was not hidden from you, when I was being made in secret, intricately woven in the depths of the earth. Your eyes saw my unformed substance; in your book were written, every one of them, the days that were formed for me, when as yet there was none of them (Psalm 139 13-16).

Every good gift and every perfect gift is from above, coming down from the Father of lights with whom there is no variation or shadow due to change (James 1:17).

"But you—you serve your GOD and He'll bless your food and your water. I'll get rid of the sickness among you; there won't be any miscarriages nor barren women in your land. I'll make sure you live full and complete lives (Exodus 23:25-26 MSG).

Prayer for a Redeemed, Supernatural Pregnancy, Labor, and Delivery

Father, we ask You in Jesus's Name for a redeemed pregnancy, labor, and delivery. We trust You for a full-term pregnancy with no miscarriage. We ask that our baby come forth at just the right time on Your chosen day. We thank You for freedom from sickness, pain, and complications.

A few verses to consider:

Then he went to the spring of water and threw salt in it and said, "Thus says the LORD, I have healed this water; from now on neither death nor miscarriage shall come from it" (2 Kings 2:21, emphasis mine).

But when the fullness of time had come, God sent forth his Son, born of woman, born under the law, to redeem those who were under the law, so that we might receive adoption as sons (Galatians 4:4-5).

Prayer for Protection and Freedom from Fear

Father, we ask for your complete protection over us, our baby, and all aspects of this pregnancy. We thank You we do not need to fear anything. Thank you in Jesus's Name for Your angels and Your loving care.

Psalm 91 is a wonderful Psalm to read as a personalized prayer. It encourages your faith in God as a wonderful Protector from evil.

Psalm 91

*He who dwells in the shelter of the Most High will abide
in the shadow of the Almighty.*

I will say to the LORD, "My refuge and my fortress, my God, in whom I trust."

For he will deliver you from the snare of the fowler and from the deadly pestilence.

*He will cover you with his pinions, and under his wings you will find refuge;
his faithfulness is a shield and buckler.*

You will not fear the terror of the night, nor the arrow that flies by day,

nor the pestilence that stalks in darkness, nor the destruction that wastes at noonday.

*A thousand may fall at your side, ten thousand at your right hand,
but it will not come near you.*

You will only look with your eyes and see the recompense of the wicked.

*Because you have made the LORD your dwelling place—
the Most High, who is my refuge*

no evil shall be allowed to befall you, no plague come near your tent.

For he will command his angels concerning you to guard you in all your ways.

On their hands they will bear you up, lest you strike your foot against a stone.

*You will tread on the lion and the adder; the young lion and
the serpent you will trample underfoot.*

*"Because he holds fast to me in love, I will deliver him;
I will protect him, because he knows my name.*

*When he calls to me, I will answer him; I will be with him in trouble;
I will rescue him and honor him.*

With long life I will satisfy him and show him my salvation."

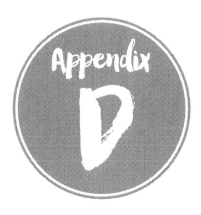

Helpful Resources

The Bible is your best resource when it comes to strengthening your faith in God's love, power, and willingness to heal. I have cited various Scriptures throughout the chapters, but here I highlight some of those and others, too. These are for you to read, meditate on, and confess out loud as you prepare to become a mother and father. Feel free to use a version that is best for you. These are from the ESV Bible. While I have listed individual verses for the sake of space, always read verses in the context of the paragraph or chapter. Be sure to write out your favorite ones and read them daily. This is one of the best ways to strengthen your faith in God and to know His desire is to heal you and bless you with a child.

Scriptures

Following are numerous Scriptures on various topics about fertility and related issues.

God's Will is Fruitful Multiplication!

So God created man in his own image, in the image of God he created him; male and female he created them. And God blessed them. And God said to them, "Be fruitful and multiply and fill the earth and subdue it, and have dominion over the fish of the sea and over the birds of the heavens and over every living thing that moves on the earth" (Genesis 1:27-28).

And God blessed Noah and his sons, and said unto them, Be fruitful, and, multiply and replenish the earth (Genesis 9:1).

And you, be fruitful and multiply increase greatly on the earth and multiply in it (Genesis 9:7).

The angel of the Lord also said to her, "I will surely multiply your offspring so that they cannot be numbered for multitude" (Genesis 16:10).

As for Ishmael, I have heard you; behold, I have blessed him and will make him fruitful and multiply him greatly. He shall father twelve princes, and I will make him into a great nation (Genesis 17:20).

I will surely bless you, and I will surely multiply your offspring as the stars of heaven and as the sand that is on the seashore. And your offspring shall possess the gate of his enemies . . . (Genesis 22:17).

I will multiply your offspring as the stars of heaven and will give to your offspring all these lands. And in your offspring all the nations of the earth shall be blessed . . . (Genesis 26:4).

And the Lord appeared to him the same night and said, "I am the God of Abraham your father. Fear not, for I am with you and will bless you and multiply your offspring for my servant Abraham's sake" (Genesis 26:24).

God Almighty bless you and make you fruitful and multiply you, that you may become a company of peoples (Genesis 28:3).

And God said to him, "I am God Almighty: be fruitful and multiply. A nation and a company of nations shall come from you, and kings shall come from your own body" (Genesis 35:11).

"Behold, I will make you fruitful and multiply, and I will make of you a company of peoples and will give this land to your offspring after you for an everlasting possession" (Genesis 48:4).

Remember Abraham, Isaac, and Israel, your servants, to whom you swore by your own self, and said to them, "I will multiply your offspring as the stars of heaven, and all this land that I have promised I will give to your offspring, and they shall inherit it forever" (Exodus 32:13).

I will turn to you and make you fruitful and multiply you and will confirm my covenant with you (Leviticus 26:9).

Hear therefore, O Israel, and be careful to do them, that it may go well with you, and that you may multiply greatly, as the Lord the God of your fathers, has promised you, in a land flowing with milk and honey (Deuteronomy 6:3).

He will love you, bless you, and multiply you. He will also bless the fruit of your womb and the fruit of your ground, your grain and your wine and your oil, the increase of your herds and the young of your flock, in the land that he swore to your fathers to give you (Deuteronomy 7:13).

The whole commandment that I command you today you shall be careful to do, that you may live and multiply and go in and possess the land that the Lord swore to give to your fathers (Deuteronomy 8:1).

None of the devoted things shall stick to your hand, that the Lord may turn from the fierceness of his anger and show you mercy and have compassion on you and multiply you, as he swore to your fathers . . . (Deuteronomy 13:17).

If you obey the commandments of the Lord your God that I command you today, by loving the Lord your God, by walking in his ways, and by keeping his commandments and his statutes and his rules, then you shall live and multiply, and the Lord, your God will bless you in the land that you are entering to take possession of it (Deuteronomy 30:16).

By his blessing they multiply greatly, and he does not let their livestock diminish (Psalm 107:38).

Behold, children are a heritage from the Lord, the fruit of the womb a reward. Like arrows in the hand of a warrior are the children of one's youth. Blessed is the man who fills his quiver with them! He shall not be put to shame when he speaks with his enemies in the gate (Psalm 127:3-5).

Look to Abraham your father and to Sarah who bore you; for he was but one when I called him, that I might bless him and multiply him (Isaiah 51:2).

Then I will gather the remnant of my flock out of all the countries where I have driven them, and I will bring them back to their fold, and they shall be fruitful and multiply (Jeremiah 23:3).

Take wives and have sons and daughters; take wives for your sons, and give your daughters in marriage, that they may bear sons and daughters; multiply there, and do not decrease (Jeremiah 29:6).

Out of them shall come songs of thanksgiving, and the voices of those who celebrate. I will multiply them, and they shall not be few; I will make them honored, and they shall not be small (Jeremiah 30:19).

As the host of heaven cannot be numbered and the sands of the sea cannot be measured, so I will multiply the offspring of David my servant, and the Levitical priests who minister to me (Jeremiah 33:22).

I will make a covenant of peace with them. It shall be an everlasting covenant with them. And I will set them in their land and multiply them, and will set my sanctuary in their midst forevermore (Ezekiel 37:26).

Surely I will bless you and multiply you (Hebrews 6:14).

NOTE: Be sure to read the entire stories of these accounts!   Be inspired and encouraged. Our God is a God of fruitful multiplication for sure!

God Heals Barrenness

And Isaac prayed to the Lord for his wife, because she was barren. And the Lord granted his prayer, and Rebekah his wife conceived (Genesis 25:21).

When the Lord saw that Leah was hated, he opened her womb, but Rachel was barren (Genesis 29:31).

None shall miscarry or be barren in your land; I will fulfill the number of your days (Exodus 23:26).

He will love you, bless you, and multiply you. He will also bless the fruit of your womb and the fruit of your ground, your grain and your wine and your oil, the increase of your herds and the young of your flock, in the land that he swore to your fathers to give you. You shall be blessed above all peoples. There shall not be male or female barren among you or among your livestock (Deuteronomy 7:13-14).

And the angel of the Lord appeared to the woman and said to her, "Behold, you are barren and have not borne children, but you shall conceive and bear a son" (Judges 13:3).

And the angel of the Lord appeared to the woman and said to her, "Behold, you are barren and have not borne children, but you shall conceive and bear a son" (1 Samuel 2:5).

He gives the barren woman a home, making her the joyous mother of children. Praise the Lord! (Psalm 113:9).

"Sing, O barren one, who did not bear; break forth into singing and cry aloud, you who have not been in labor! For the children of the desolate one will be more than the children of her who is married," says the Lord (Isaiah 54:1).

And behold, your relative Elizabeth in her old age has also conceived a son, and this is the sixth month with her who was called barren (Luke 1:36).

For it is written, "Rejoice, O barren one who does not bear; break forth and cry aloud, you who are not in labor! For the children of the desolate one will be more than those of the one who has a husband" (Galatians 4:27).

NOTE: Rejoice O Barren Woman! There is hope and healing for you.

God's Will is Healing and Health

Then Abraham prayed to God, and God healed Abimelech, and also healed his wife and female slaves so that they bore children (Genesis 20:17).

O Lord my God, I cried to You for help, and You have healed me (Psalm 30:2).

Bless the Lord O my soul, and forget not all His benefits, who forgives all your iniquity, who heals all your diseases . . . (Psalm 103:1).

He sent out His word and healed them, and delivered them from their destruction (Psalm 107:20).

But He was pierced for our transgressions; He was crushed for our iniquities; upon Him was the chastisement that brought us peace, and with His wounds we are healed (Isaiah 53:5).

Heal me, O Lord and I shall be healed; save me, and I shall be saved, for You are my praise (Jeremiah 17:14).

So his fame spread throughout all Syria, and they brought Him all the sick, those afflicted with various diseases and pains, those oppressed by demons, epileptics, and paralytics, and He healed them (Matthew 4:24).

When He went ashore He saw a great crowd, and He had compassion on them and healed their sick (Matthew 14:14).

And immediately the flow of blood dried up, and she felt in her body that she was healed of her disease (Mark 5:29).

But now even more the report about Him went abroad, and great crowds gathered to hear Him and to be healed of their infirmities (Luke 5:15).

The people also gathered from the towns around Jerusalem, bringing the sick and those afflicted with unclean spirits, and they were all healed (Acts 5:16).

Therefore, confess your sins to one another and pray for one another, that you may be healed. The prayer of a righteous person has great power as it is working (James 5:16).

NOTE: There are so many more passages on healing! Please do your own study and watch your faith in the Great Physician, Jesus, grow!

God Answers Prayer

"Ask, and it will be given to you; seek, and you will find; knock, and it will be opened to you. For everyone who asks receives, and the one who seeks finds, and to the one who knocks it will be opened. Or which one of you, if his son asks him for bread, will give him a stone? Or if he asks for a fish, will give him a serpent? If you then, who are evil, know how to give good gifts to your children, how much more will your Father who is in heaven give good things to those who ask him!" (Matthew 7:7-11).

And whatever you ask in prayer you will receive, if you have faith (Matthew 21:22).

Therefore I tell you, whatever you ask in prayer believe that you have received it, and it will be yours (Mark 11:24).

But the angel said to him, "Do not be afraid, Zechariah, for your prayer has been heard, and your wife Elizabeth will bear you a son, and you shall call his name John" (Luke 1:13).

Do not be anxious about anything, but in everything by prayer and supplication with thanksgiving let your requests be made known to God (Philippians 4:6).

And the prayer of faith will save the one who is sick, and the Lord will raise him up. And if he has committed sins, he will be forgiven. Therefore, confess your sins to one another and pray for one another, that you may be healed. The prayer of a righteous person has great power as it is working (James 5:15-16).

And this is the confidence that we have toward Him, that if we ask anything according to His will He hears us. And if we know that He hears us in whatever we ask, we know that we have the requests that we have asked of Him (1 John 5:14-15).

NOTE: Again, do your own study on prayer. It will amaze you how eager and faithful God is to answer prayer!

God Loves You

See what kind of love the Father has given to us, that we should be called children of God; and so we are. The reason why the world does not know us is that it did not know Him (1 John 3:1).

So we have come to know and to believe the love that God has for us. God is love, and whoever abides in love abides in God, and God abides in him.

By this is love perfected with us, so that we may have confidence for the Day of Judgment, because as He is so also are we in this world. There is no fear in love, but perfect love casts out fear. For fear has to do with punishment, and whoever fears has not been perfected in love (1 John 4:16-18).

In that day you will ask in my name, and I do not say to you that I will ask the Father on your behalf; for the Father himself loves you, because you have loved me and have believed that I came from God (John 16:26).

No, in all these things we are more than conquerors through Him who loved us. For I am sure that neither death nor life, nor angels nor rulers, nor things present nor things to come, nor powers, nor height nor depth, nor anything else in all creation, will be able to separate us from the love of God in Christ Jesus our Lord (Romans 8:37-39).

NOTE: The Bible overflows with verses about God's love. Soak in them!

Books

I love books! My life has been transformed through reading. I could recommend hundreds of books on these topics but will refrain. I do not agree with everything that is in all of these books, but read them with the Holy Spirit, and He will show you what's important for you and your journey.

The Gospel

You may think you already know the Good News of Jesus Christ. However, as a pastor, I have found many people are genuinely confused or have been taught half-truths about Jesus and His finished work on the Cross. The following resources will open your eyes to the glorious Gospel of our Lord Jesus Christ. Be prepared to be set free and fall in love with Jesus all over again. This will change your life more than having children.

- *The Gospel in Ten Words* by Paul Ellis
- *Grace Walk* by Steve McVey
- *Mystical Union* by John Crowder

God's Character

It is so important that you know your Father is a good, loving Father who wants to give you good things. Read these and be convinced!

- *The Good and Beautiful God* by James B. Smith
- *Destined to Reign* by Joseph Prince
- *He Loves Me: Learning to Live in the Father's Affection by* Wayne Jacobsen
- *The Shack* by William Paul Young

The Holy Spirit

I have included a few books about the Holy Spirit because He is the whole reason I am a mother today! After I was filled with the Spirit, I saw God's will was healing, and the rest is history. I love you, Holy Spirit!

- *Baptism in the Holy Spirit* by Randy Clark
- *The New You and the Holy Spirit* by Andrew Wommack
- *Hello, Holy Spirit: God's Gift of Live-In Help* by Dianne Leman (to be published in 2017)

Healing

There are many good books on this topic. My favorite book, though, is the Bible itself. When you read the accounts of Jesus healing so many people, you will be convinced that healing is God's will. Here are a couple others to help convince you!

- *Essential Guide to Healing* by Randy Cark and Bill Johnson
- *Power Healing* by John Wimber
- *Doing Healing* by Alexander Venter

Prophetic

Prophecy is one of the gifts of the Holy Spirit that is for everyone! This gift is so valuable as you listen for God's encouragement. All can learn to give and receive prophecy.

- *Translating God* by Shawn Bolz
- *Developing Your Prophetic Gifting* by Graham Cooke

Childbirth

I am a strong advocate for a redeemed pregnancy, labor, and delivery. In other words, I believe Jesus wants us to have a pain-free, nausea-free, complication-free experience. I do not agree with everything in these books, but I do agree with a natural, Christ-centered pregnancy and birth.

- *Supernatural Childbirth* by Jackie Mize
- *Handbook for Christian Natural Birth* by Marianne Manley
- *Ina May's Guide to Childbirth* by Ina May Gaskin

Prayer

These books help you learn how to pray in faith. Very good, especially if you have had poor teaching on prayer in the past.

- *A Better Way to Pray* by Andrew Wommack
- *Lord, Teach Us To Pray* by Andrew Murray
- *A Praying Life: Connecting with God in a Distracting World* by Paul Miller

Prayers for Pregnancy

Amazon lists numerous books. Choose the best one for you! Or better yet, write your own prayers and read them aloud daily to remind you of your Father's goodness, love, and gift of children.

- *Praying Through Your Pregnancy: An Inspirational Week-by-Week Guide for Bonding with Your Baby* by Jennifer Polimina and Carolyn Warren
- *Expecting: Praying for Your Child's Development—Body and Soul* by Marla Taviano

Marriage

Books alone cannot make a good marriage, but there are some very good resources that will strengthen your marriage.

- *The Five Love Languages: The Secret to Love that Lasts* by Gary Chapman
- *Intended for Pleasure: Sex Technique and Sexual Fulfillment in Christian Marriage* by Ed Wheat
- *The Seven Principles for Making Marriage Work: A Practical Guide from the Country's Foremost Relationship Expert* by John Gottman

Parenting

There are many great books on parenting. We have a very distinct style that we embrace—probably a bit more old-fashioned than most. But all of our children love Jesus and have grown into responsible adults. So, we heartily recommend these!

- *The New Six-Point Plan for Raising Happy, Healthy Children* by John Rosemond (I noticed on Amazon that Rosemond has many newer books. Check them out!)
- *Reaching the Heart of Your Teen* by Gary Ezzo
- *Loving Our Kids on Purpose: Making a Heart to Heart Connection* by Danny Silk

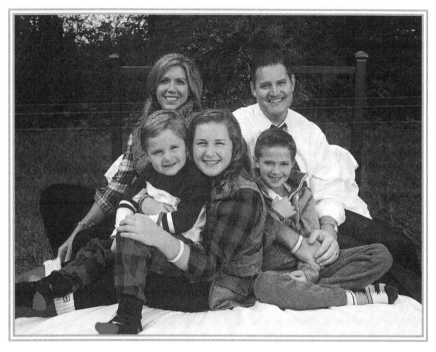

Dawn, Rich, Graycen, Faith and Luke Daugherty.

Worship

Loving God with all my being has changed my life! Worship is so powerful and releases faith and love in our hearts. There are so many great worship recordings now, so choose what is best for you to express your love to Jesus and receive His love in return. Personal favorites of mine:

- Vineyard Worship Music
- Bethel Music
- Hillsong United
- Jesus Culture

Acknowledgments

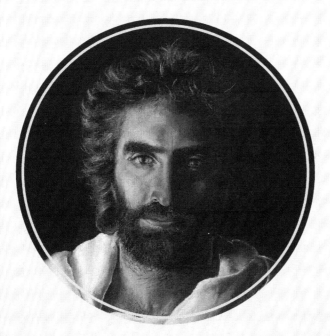

"Prince of Peace" by Akiane

I will thank you, Lord, among all the people.
I will sing your praises among the nations.
For your unfailing love is higher than the heavens.
Your faithfulness reaches to the clouds.

Be exalted, O God, above the highest heavens.
May your glory shine over all the earth (Psalm 108:3-5).

Acknowledgments

First and foremost, I thank God, my amazing Father, who gives us the incredible privilege of having children. Your love and faithfulness astound me every day. Thank You for making it possible for us to overcome the pain and impossibility of infertility and for us to experience all the joy (and sorrow!) of parenthood. Thank You for sending Jesus to right the wrongs of our lives and thank You for the most precious gift of the Holy Spirit, who opens our hearts and heals our bodies.

I thank my wonderful life partner and husband of 45 years, Happy. You have not only traveled the path of infertility with me, but you have also been my perfect partner in parenting our five beautiful children, pastoring our amazing church, and now together, making lifetime memories as Papa Hap and Manna Di with our growing brood of special grandchildren. You have been my greatest encourager in writing this book, and I could not have done it without you. Silver Fox, I love you with all my heart!

Thank you to all the women and men who over the many years have been willing to pray with couples who were battling infertility. Thank you for sacrificing many hours to gather, pray, and pray again. Thank you for weeping and rejoicing as we witnessed God's miracles over and over. Thank you that you continue to pray for those couples who are still waiting for their miracle. Special thanks to Gayle Wildman, Doral Johnson, Judy Swartzendruber, Julie Yoder, and Dawn Daugherty. You are all true champions for the infertile couples.

A big thank you to Katie Goulet, who designed this beautiful cover, did the photography, and also oversees my website and Facebook page. Katie is also the blessed recipient of God's cure for infertility. She now joyfully raises three sons along with her hubby, Daniel, our gifted worship leader at The Vineyard Church and one of my greatest encouragers.

I was so excited that Katie Hart and her hubby Brad agreed to be the models for the cover because they, like many of you, struggled with infertility. They are now the very blessed and busy parents of three wonderful sons and a beautiful daughter. Thank you, Katie and Brad!

Thank you to my brother, Tim Hoerr, and his wife Toni, whose generosity made this book possible. You gave us your Coronado condo so I could write unhindered and you gave in so many other ways that made all the difference to me. I love you both.

Thank you to Melissa Logsdon, Nicole Milt, and my daughter-in-law, Jenna Leman, who all faithfully edited this manuscript while still waiting for their miracles. That was not easy! I can't wait to rejoice with each of you.

Thank you to Teresa Meacham, who also brilliantly edited this manuscript while awaiting the birth of twins who were the answer to many prayers after many tears. Your heartfelt input was invaluable!

My longtime friends Burnsey Eisenmenger and Ruthie Wegman both gave me such great help with their fantastic grammar skills and mastery of the English language. But most of all, Burnsey and Ruthie, I so appreciated your encouragement and friendship in the writing process.

Of course, I am also indebted to the men who were willing to tackle this project: particularly Tom Burtness and Don Follis, who gave me their writing expertise and a much-needed male perspective. You guys are both gifted writers and I thank you for your help.

My "real" editor, Tom Hanlon, is a rare gem. He not only gave superb editing, but he also knew my heart, my faith, my life, and was such a valuable asset to seeing this project through. Thank you, Tom!

I could never have written this book without the help of all the women and men who were willing to share their miraculous stories of God's cure for their infertility and the blessing of children in their lives. Thank you for baring your hearts, and being willing to let others learn and be encouraged through your stories. I especially thank my own daughter, Julie Yoder, who battled infertility with her husband Mike and now is the most blessed mom of three, our precious grandchildren, of course!

Last, but certainly not least, I thank our incredible family: J.D. and Carrie Leman, A.J. and Kim Leman, Mike and Julie Yoder, J and Katy Leman, Cory and Jenna Leman, and our fast-growing gang of gregarious grands. You are all God's reminder to me every day that our God, your God, is a God of the Impossible! He is a God who delights in families. He is a God whose unfailing love is higher than the heavens and whose faithfulness reaches to the clouds. He is a God who is still blessing couples with babies and the indescribable joy of family. My heart overflows with love for all of you. My prayers for you will never stop. My joy is unspeakable. All of you know, "This is the day the Lord has made, I will rejoice and be glad in it!"

I have always thought *Acknowledgments* in a book were a bit over the top and not that important or necessary. However, as I sat writing this today, I saw how wrong I was. It is actually true that "It takes a village to write a book!" This has definitely been my experience and I am deeply grateful to all who have contributed, helped, and encouraged in ways I cannot even begin to acknowledge. Our wonderful, supportive church family, the precious people of The Vineyard Church of Central Illinois, have loved me, listened to me, helped me, prayed for me, and made it possible for me to be the woman I am today. It is such a joy to do life with a community of people who radically love Jesus and unashamedly welcome the Presence of the Holy Spirit!

With love and thankfulness,

Di

72060414R00115

Made in the USA
Columbia, SC
14 June 2017